Stories of Intensive Care
Medical Challenges and Ethical Dilemmas in Real Patients

Lawrence Martin, M.D.
Clinical Professor of Medicine (retired)
Case Western Reserve University School of Medicine, Cleveland
drlarry437@gmail.com

Pictures and Drawings

Line drawings in "The Yellow Man" and "Thyroid Storm" by Dan Traynor

Time Magazine cover in "Too Much Sugar" from:
http://content.time.com/time/covers/0,16641,19230827,00.html

News item on 1923 Nobel Prize in "Too Much Sugar" from:
https://www.pinterest.com/pin/858217272716971984/

Discovers of Insulin in "Too Much Sugar" from:
https://bantinghousenhsc.wordpress.com/2015/12/06/banting-and-best-and-macleod-and-collip/

Artist's depiction of Dickens' Fat Boy Joe in "Pickwickian," drawing of endotracheal tube in "Extraordinary Care," chest x-rays in "Adult Respiratory Distress," and AED pictures in "Shock Him!," are from Wikimedia Commons: https://commons.wikimedia.org/wiki/

Book cover in "The Red Baron" from https://books2read.com/u/meBwgE
Movie poster in "The Red Baron" from
https://www.imdb.com/title/tt0096764/?ref_=fn_al_tt_2

Photograph of peak flow meter in "Rounds," and EKG tracings in "Shock Him!," are from the author.

***

ISBN: 978-0-9978959-5-7

Published 2020
Lakeside Press
The Villages, FL

DEDICATION:

To all the staff who worked with me at Cleveland's
Mt. Sinai Hospital, 1976–2000

The following stories were originally published as magazine articles.

"Adult Respiratory Distress" as "A Case for Intensive Care," in *The Gamut*, Fall 1982

"Crusade" as "Hammer Home the Message to Patients Who Smoke," in *Medical Economics*, January 1991

"Pickwickian," in *The Gamut*, Winter 1991

"We can't kill your mother!" in *Medical Economics*, March 1991

"Extraordinary Care" as "Mr. Bowman's Solution," in *The Saturday Evening Post*, April 1991

"Too Much Sugar, Too Little History" in *The Gamut*, Winter, 1992

"The Red Baron" in *The Saturday Evening Post*, January 1993

"Mommy, why don't you hug me?" in *The Saturday Evening Post*, May 1993.

"The Wild Man" in *The Saturday Evening Post*, October 1994

"Call NASA!" in *Resident & Staff Physician*, July 1995

"'Lou Gehrig' Strikes Again" in *The Saturday Evening Post*, July 1995

"Shock Him!" in *The Saturday Evening Post*, June 1996

Stories of Intensive Care

Medical Challenges and Ethical Dilemmas in Real Patients

Table of Contents

Preface

Who is this book for?

This is the second edition of a book that first came out in 2001. Then it was titled *"We Can't Kill Your Mother!" and Other Stories of Intensive Care*. The stories have been updated where necessary, to put in perspective medical care that was provided back in the 1980s and 1990s. All the patients were cared for in Cleveland's Mt. Sinai Hospital.

Technology has improved since then, and we have many new medications, but of course the diseases, the end-of-life ethical dilemmas, and how people react to illness have not changed. Thus, these stories are as timely now as when first published.

Many of these stories were originally published in lay periodicals, including *The Saturday Evening Post*. While I have also written several medical textbooks, in preparing these stories I put on a different writer's hat—that of a physician whose goal is to explain medical and ethical situations to the general reader.

No special background or medical expertise is necessary to enjoy or understand these stories. In fact, the only "requirement" is an interest in humanity. Illness and medicine are universal, and everyone has some familiarity with hospitals, if only from the position of a consumer. Most people have, at some point, either been hospitalized or visited a friend or family member in the hospital. These stories take you inside the medical intensive care unit, a major part of every acute care hospital. That's the setting, but the subject is people and their serious—and sometimes strange—afflictions.

Who are the patients?

The stories are based on real patients cared for in the medical intensive care unit (MICU) of Mt. Sinai Hospital, at one time a major Cleveland teaching hospital. For many years, our hospital had the best statistics in the region for ICU mortality. Sadly, the hospital closed its doors in February 2000, a victim of changing demographics and other factors. However, all these patients were cared for when the hospital was thriving, and thus frequent use is made of the present tense. To preserve patient anonymity, all names have been changed, as well as some of the descriptive details.

The first chapter gives an overview of intensive care rounds and how the MICU operates. Succeeding chapters are devoted to one or two patients and the challenges they present. Like Harold Switek, too ill to leave MICU, too psychotic to stay. And Willie the Yellow Man, whose love affair with alcohol exceeded anything you've ever seen. You'll meet a young socialite hospitalized with rapid onset of total paralysis and wonder (as we did): will she ever hug her kids again? And another woman about to have her baby during a terrifying asthma attack. Then there's the young accountant who slept in a coma—for six months! In "The Red Baron" I tell the strange saga of a man who claimed to be coughing up blood, only that wasn't his real problem.

As in most hospitals today, in Mt. Sinai the *medical* ICU was separate from the *surgical* intensive care unit, the latter staffed for post-operative patients and trauma victims. MICU is also separate from the *coronary* care unit, where patients are sent with heart attacks and other cardiac emergencies. Whatever the physical arrangement, every sizable hospital handles the same problems and encounters the same ethical dilemmas as presented by our patients. Like elderly, senile Mr. Zigson, who is trying to die a natural death. Only problem: he has no family. Should the doctors leave him alone or "do everything"? And the nursing home patient who is awake and alert but can only live connected to a breathing machine. Her daughter demands that the ventilator be disconnected so "Mother can die." Can doctors honor such a request? Can they *ignore* it?

Should a physician write about his or her patients?

Emphatically, yes, if he or she is so inclined and provided that privacy is maintained. In a literary sense, doctors and nurses are privileged. What we see in our daily jobs is more than enough to fill many interesting books. We just have to find the time and inclination to tell others about what we do, and to make the work seem as interesting in print as it is in real life.

Lawrence Martin, M.D.
The Villages, FL
January, 2020
drlarry437@gmail.com

1.   Rounds

"If possible, try not to use a teaching hospital during the summer months."
—Dr. Mehmet Oz

Why would the renowned cardiologist Dr. Oz write something like that? Well, it's because July is the start of a new training year: newly graduated medical students start as interns, and residents with just a year of training are now supervising the new interns. Dr. Oz goes on to compare being a patient in that period to having your transmission repaired by a neophyte mechanic. "At the very least," he recommends staying out of the hospital the first part of July.

The best advice is not to be sick enough to need a hospital, but if you are, don't worry so much about July in a teaching hospital. The advice is somewhat exaggerated. Yes, the house staff—interns and residents—are new, but they are not the only ones caring for the patient. There are senior residents, and attending physicians as well. Or there should be. That was certainly the situation at my hospital, Mt. Sinai Medical Center in Cleveland. As the director of the hospital's medical intensive care unit (MICU), it was my job to supervise and teach house staff and help manage patients admitted there.

On the first day of the new academic year, July first, I greeted the two new interns. "Welcome to MICU. I'm Dr. Martin. I run the unit and will be rounding with you this month. How does it feel to be starting your internship?"

"Scary," said Deborah Hafly, a petite, energetic woman who came to Mt. Sinai with top recommendations. She and her partner on this rotation, Michael Highland, were both excellent students and were expected to perform well as interns.

"You've met the medical resident, Jerry Clark, and been assigned your patients?"

"Yes," said Deborah. "He assigned us our patients this morning. We each have four."

"Good. Well, let's make rounds."

MICU occupies a large rectangular space on the second floor of the hospital. The "unit," as it is often referred to, consists of eight single-bed rooms arranged in a broad-based U shape, in the center of which is the nursing station. On either side of the nursing station. double doors lead to the hallway and family waiting area.

1

All the patient rooms are fronted by sliding glass doors that can be pushed open for quick access; drapes across the doors provide privacy when necessary. Each patient can be 'wired' so that his or her cardiac rhythm is continuously displayed on monitors at the nursing station.

The nurse-to-patient ratio in MICU is as high as one-to-one when every patient is critically ill. Despite the appellation 'intensive', not all MICU patients are critical. On average, when the unit is full, five nurses per shift can provide excellent care. On the regular hospital wards at Mt. Sinai, the average ratio is one registered nurse per eight patients.

MICU rounds are open to anyone on the staff who may have something to contribute. Besides the attending physician (myself or an associate), rounds include two interns, the supervising resident, one or more nurses, and a respiratory therapist. Also participating, on occasion, are medical and nursing students, various consultants and private attending physicians, and a social worker.

If Mt. Sinai was not a teaching hospital, my job would be much more difficult, perhaps impossible. Most MICU patients require constant management, something not easily done over the phone, or even during brief hospital visits. Physicians must always be available to order medications, adjust ventilator settings, put in catheters, talk to families, examine and treat new admissions, and transfer patients to the regular wards. Private, office-based physicians who send their patients to MICU are thankful for the house staff and round-the-clock physician coverage. Without interns and residents, we could not provide the excellent care Mt. Sinai's MICU is known for.

House staff, although licensed MDs, are in training and not certified in any specialty. They must be supervised throughout their three or more years of hospital internship and residency. Interns, fresh out of medical school, are supervised by the junior resident, he or she by the senior resident, and all the house staff by the chief resident, full-time staff, and visiting physicians.

Physician training is a dynamic, patient-centered process. Lectures occupy no more than an hour a day of house staff training. Most of the learning comes from supervised, hands-on patient care, supplemented by reading journals and textbooks.

* * *

I took the new interns over to Room 1, where we met Dr. Clark and the MICU head nurse.

"Let me introduce you to Marsha Ligner, MICU's head nurse," I said. "Marsha, this is Deborah Hafly and Michael Highland, our two new interns."

"Welcome to MICU," she replied. "Glad to have you aboard." Turning toward me, Marsha continued, "Dr. Martin, who can we transfer out this morning?"

"I don't know. Do we need a bed right away?"

"Yes. The ER just called. They have an overdose that needs to come up."

I turned to Dr. Clark, the medical resident. "Who can go out?"

"I just put Mr. Jones up for transfer. As soon as a bed's ready upstairs, he can go."

"Okay. Marsha, find us a bed for Mr. Jones. And please ask Patient Placement not to drag their feet. I know there are empty beds on the wards."

Marsha nodded. She would make one or two phone calls, and Mr. Jones would soon be transferred.

"Is the ER patient intubated?" I asked.

"Not as far as I know," said Dr. Clark.

"Okay. Well, let's start rounds. We'll see the new patient as soon as he arrives. Or is it she?"

"A twenty-year-old woman. She OD'd on tricyclics."

I stood with my back to the sliding glass doors of Room 1, chart rack and house staff before me. We were also joined by two of the MICU nurses and a respiratory therapist.

"Has everyone met Dr. Hafly and Dr. Highland?" Everyone had. I addressed the two interns, the only new people on the team. "We round at ten each morning. You should be up to date on your patients by the time rounds begin. Today is an exception, of course. Also, we require that you write a chart note on each of your patients every day. You need to list all their medical problems, all drugs they are receiving, and all the tubes entering or exiting their body. Dr. Clark already went over this requirement with you, didn't he?"

They nodded yes.

"Good. Jerry, why don't you briefly present each patient as we go around." Jerry Clark, 28, had been the MICU resident in June and was staying another day to orient the new interns. He knew all the patients.

"Okay," he began. "In Room One we have Mr. Hewlett Jones. He's a sixty-seven-year-old man admitted June twenty seventh, with a CVA."

"What's a CVA?" I asked Deborah.

"Cerebrovascular accident," she answered, matter-of-factly.

"Jerry, did Mr. Jones have an accident?" I wanted to send a signal early in the month: avoid jargon if possible.

Dr. Clark showed a knowing smile. He had been through this routine with me before. In the spirit of the new year he played it straight—almost.

"No, Dr. Martin," he replied, with a trace of sarcasm. "He had a stroke.

There was no accident."

"I see. Then why do you call it a cerebrovascular *accident*? Why didn't you—why don't we—just say Mr. Jones had a stroke and be done with it?"

The interns stared in mild disbelief. What kind of rounds were these? English 101? Every new doctor has heard the term "CVA" a hundred times, always indicating a stroke of some sort. Drs. Hafly and Highland had never before heard anyone *question* the term.

"I don't know," admitted Dr. Clark. "That's just what everyone calls it. I know it makes no sense."

"I agree. It's just one of those terms that gets introduced into medicine, and no one ever questions. Okay, go on."

"Well, he had a stroke, a spontaneously-occurring blood clot blocking his left middle cerebral artery. The clot paralyzed his right side and left him aphasic, but I think he's getting better. Neurology's following him, and he's ready for transfer."

We entered Mr. Jones's room to say goodbye. Reflecting the crossover of nerve pathways, the right side of his body was limp from a blockage in the left side of his brain. Since the speech center is on the left, Mr. Jones couldn't talk, but he recognized us and understood conversation. I explained that he was being transferred out of MICU, that he was improving and with continued physical therapy had an excellent prognosis for recovery. He understood. We left Mr. Jones and rolled the chart rack over to Room 2, stopping in front of the closed glass doors.

"This is Mr. Fisher," said Dr. Clark. "He's a thirty-four-year-old man admitted June twenty-ninth with a severe asthma attack. He has improved but we want to continue IV steroids and inhaled bronchodilators another day. His peak flow is up to one forty."

Through the glass, we saw a young man in mild respiratory distress, apparent by a fast breathing rate.

"Who's got Mr. Fisher?"

"Deborah."

"OK. Deborah, did you learn about peak flow in medical school?"

"I didn't have that much experience managing asthma patients. I think I only had one asthmatic on my medicine clerkship."

"Well, you'll become an expert here. Peak flow is the best single breathing test to follow the progress of an asthmatic. It takes only a few seconds and, if done properly, the test is fairly reproducible."

I asked Greg, our respiratory therapist, to get the peak flow meter so I could demonstrate the test. He went into Mr. Fisher's room and brought back a round, metal instrument the size of a small kitchen clock. A handle on the side of the peak flow meter allows the patient to hold the instrument horizontal while blowing into a mouthpiece situated above the handle. A long needle on the face of the meter deflects when air is blown into the mouthpiece; the harder the blow, the greater the deflection. A slight 'puff' into the mouthpiece by a normal adult will register at least 150 liters/minute peak flow. A maximal effort will register at least 400 liters/minute.

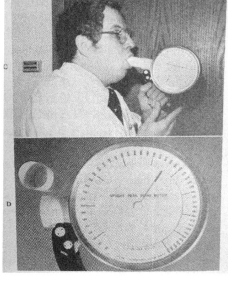

The photo shows the peak flow needle at zero before the maneuver and at 550 liters/minute afterwards.

I inserted a cardboard mouthpiece into the meter and handed it to Deborah. "Deborah, just put your lips around the mouth-piece and give a little puff." She did as instructed, and the needle deflected to 180.

"Now reset the needle and take a deep breath, then blow out with all your strength." The needle went to 495.

"Okay, now let's go see our patient."

Mr. Fisher sat in his bed, appearing physically strong but humbled by his asthma.

"How do you feel?" I asked. "Are you any better since you've come in?"

"Oh, much better," he said, with conviction.

But how much better was he? You can be fooled by patients. A 30 percent improvement from a severe asthma attack can make the patient feel like a million bucks, at least at rest. He was still breathing faster than normal, and I heard wheezing on exam.

I inserted a fresh mouthpiece and asked Mr. Fisher to do the peak flow maneuver. He took in a deep breath and blew as hard as he could: 170. I asked him to repeat the effort. The needle went to 168.

"Well, you still have a way to go. Your peak flow is still reduced. We're going to keep you here today and continue the intravenous medication. You might be able to leave the ICU tomorrow." I thanked him, and we stepped outside.

"What do you think?" I asked the interns.

"I'm surprised," said Dr. Highland. "He doesn't look that short of breath."

"I agree. I think he may have chronic asthma. The only way to gauge severity of asthma is with the peak flow or some similar measurement. Despite maximal effort he couldn't get above 170 on the peak flow." I looked at Deborah. "You did better than that with almost no effort. He looks strong, but if he ran a race with you right now, it would be no contest."

"What's going to happen to him?" asked Deborah.

"Too soon to tell," I replied. "He's much better than yesterday, that's for sure. If he can't reach a higher peak flow despite several more days of IV therapy, then his impairment is chronic. He used to smoke heavily, so that may be contributing. Anyway, it's too early to say. We'll watch him in MICU one more day, then send him upstairs if he remains stable."

We moved to Room 3. "This is Mr. Denton Smith," said Dr. Clark. "He came in last night with a gastrointestinal hemorrhage. He's a heavy alcoholic. GI's already 'scoped' him."

"What'd they find?" The gastroenterology service is good at putting "scopes," long flexible tubes with a light on the end and a channel through the middle, into the stomach of bleeding patients.

"A large duodenal ulcer. Here's a picture."

Dr. Clark opened up the chart. Taped in the middle of a progress note was an amazingly sharp, digitized photo of an intestinal ulcer. In the middle of a normal stomach lining sat a white dime-sized patch, and, in the middle of that, a tiny dab of red. I read the handwritten legend under the photo. "Eroding gastric ulcer with bleeding vessel as shown. Vessel cauterized."

"Has his bleeding stopped?"

"Yes, but GI wants us to observe him for another day. We've given him a total of three units of blood."

"Okay. I see in the note that he has continued to drink. Was he drunk when he came in?"

"No, he says he hasn't had anything to drink in three days. So we're also going to watch for DTs [delirium tremens]."

"Didn't anyone ever tell him to quit drinking?" I asked. It was a rhetorical question. "What's his hematocrit?"

"It was only 23 percent on admission. After the three units it's up to 30." (Normal for a man is 40 percent – 46 percent.)

Suddenly two nurses from the station began running toward Room 7. The first to arrive punched open the door, and the other one hauled in the red crash cart. We arrived seconds later. The patient was Mrs. Waldstein, a 76-year-old woman with end-stage kidney and heart disease. The day before, she had received a shunt in her right arm for kidney dialysis. We had spent considerable time with her and her family discussing such issues as quality of life, what she could expect with dialysis, possible therapy without it, and so on. In the end she said she wasn't ready to die or become a vegetable, and accepted dialysis.

Even so, her kidney doctor was concerned about whether her heart was strong enough to withstand three times a week dialysis. She had suffered two heart attacks in the past year. Two days earlier, she was admitted to MICU with pulmonary edema from kidney and heart failure. Now her heart had suddenly stopped beating altogether. If we did nothing in the next two minutes, she would be dead.

Resuscitation is always a cacophony of orders, and this one was no different.

"Ambu bag!"

"Epinephrine!"

"Call anesthesiology!"

"They're called."

"Get the EKG. Let's get a rhythm strip."

Dr. Clark positioned himself at the head of the bed and began ventilating Mrs. Waldstein with an Ambu bag, while I took up chest compressions. One of the nurses began infusing epinephrine into an arm vein while another stuck the patient's femoral artery for a blood gas sample.

After one minute it was time to check if there was a heartbeat. My chest-pumping effort was creating an artificial heartbeat, which could mask the patient's own.

"I'll stop for just a few seconds to check the monitor," I said.

"Still flat line, Dr. Martin."

"Okay," I replied, "let's give an amp of calcium." The nurse handling drugs infused the calcium.

"Now give an amp of bicarbonate. She's acidotic from her renal failure. Somebody please listen to her chest." Deborah complied.

"Good breath sounds when Jerry's bagging," she said.

Then one of the nurses: "Dr. Martin, we've got a rhythm. Looks idioventricular."

"Any pulse?"

"Only when you pump. Can you stop for a minute?"

"Impossible. A minute is eternity." I stopped for four seconds.

"I feel something," said the nurse. "Let me check her blood pressure."

7

The anesthesiologist arrived. Good, I thought, it's Josh; he's one of the best. Anesthesiologists are expert at intubating patients, so we always call them for a cardiopulmonary arrest. By now, there were at least seven people in the room.

Josh went to the head of her bed.

"Hold off intubating for a second, Josh," I said. "Let me see what her rhythm is."

"If she's got a pressure, you still want her intubated?" he asked.

"Yes. I want to make sure she's adequately oxygenated and ventilated. This can happen again. What's her blood pressure?"

"I'm getting ninety by palpation," said the nurse. "Do you still want epi to run in?"

"Yes. Now, let's get her intubated."

Josh expertly slipped the foot-long tube into Mrs. Waldstein's throat. Seconds later, I resumed chest compressions. Dr. Clark re-started his bag breathing, only now he was pumping fresh air through the endotracheal tube, a direct conduit into her lungs.

"Looks like a nodal rhythm, Dr. Martin," said the nurse checking the monitor.

"Good. I'll stop pumping." I checked for a pulse in her groin and felt a repetitive thump against my fingertips. "Looks like she's gonna make it. Let's get a ventilator hooked up and also another blood gas. Stop the epinephrine."

We stayed in Mrs. Waldstein's room another twenty minutes, to make sure she was stable. The nurses' initial response to the cardiac arrest was so quick I doubted she had suffered any brain damage.

* * *

On leaving Mrs. Waldstein's room I noted that Deborah and Michael were staring rather idly at the cardiac monitor, Michael with his hands in his pockets. No doubt they felt insecure in the midst of this emergency and I sought to reassure them.

"Don't worry. By the end of the month you'll know exactly what to do. I promise." Affecting nonchalance, I added, "Let's resume rounds." We moved on to Room 4.

"This is John Popola," said Dr. Clark. "He's seventy-two, with end-stage Alzheimer's. He was sent here for pneumonia and respiratory failure. His sputum culture's growing *pseudomonas aeruginosa*. We have him on gentamicin and piperacillin. We can't get him off the ventilator until his pneumonia clears. He's DNR."

Before us was a man looking perhaps ten years older than seventy-two, white hair, face grizzly, eyes sunken in. He was not awake, an effect of sedation given to relieve respiratory distress.

"Deborah, Michael, you two know what DNR means, I assume."

"Do not resuscitate," said Deborah.

"Right. So, why's he connected to a life support ventilator?" I asked. There was no answer.

"Jerry, if Mr. Popola is 'Do Not Resuscitate,' why the ventilator? Isn't that a form of resuscitation?"

"He wasn't DNR until after he was intubated. Then the family decided they didn't want any more heroics. They don't want him resuscitated again if his heart stops or he crashes. So, we made him DNR."

"What family?" I asked.

"His wife is deceased. We talked to a sister and his son. They both agreed."

"Michael, how does being DNR affect the care of a ventilator patient?" This was not a fair question for the first day of internship, but I wanted the interns to think about it anyway.

"I don't know," he said.

"It just means we don't add more life support," I explained. "Otherwise, it doesn't affect the care at all. We'll treat Mr. Popola's pneumonia in the usual way, and will do our best to get him safely off the ventilator. In some circumstances, no treatment may be given a DNR patient, but that's not the case with Mr. Popola. His pneumonia is a treatable condition and may respond to antibiotics."

"Does the family have to sign for DNR status at Mt. Sinai?" Michael asked.

"No. You just have to write a note in the chart documenting that you talked to the patient if he's competent, or to the family if the patient is not."

We reviewed the ventilator settings and blood gases, then all of Mr. Popola's medications. There was still a way to go before he could breathe unassisted by the machine. We moved on.

"In Room 5 we have Elsie McKnight," Dr. Clark said. "She's a Tylenol overdose."

"Looks like a young woman to me," I said. At that, Dr. Clark rolled his eyes and made a here-we-go-again face.

I ignored him and addressed the interns. "Suppose a patient pointed to you and said, 'There's a stethoscope,' or 'here we have a reflex hammer.'"

"Okay, okay," Dr. Clark said, in a manner of 'enough, enough'. Actually, he took my comments good-naturedly. They were really intended to impress the interns and, perhaps, change in some minuscule way the language of medicine. Doctors already well into their post-graduate training, like Dr. Clark, were usually beyond my message.

Dr. Clark resumed his patient report, facing the two interns. "Miss McKnight is a twenty-five-year-old woman who *took* an overdose of Tylenol tablets. When she came to the ER, they measured her acetaminophen [Tylenol] level. It was twenty-four."

"Michael, do you have any question about that?" I asked. "What would you want to know at that point?"

"Was she breathing?"

"No, I don't mean about her vital signs. Obviously, you want to know if a patient is breathing, if her heart is beating, and so forth. I mean, given that she took Tylenol and you have a blood level of the drug, what specific question should you ask?"

Michael thought for a moment. "What else did she take?"

"Well, that's important too, but let's assume it's only Tylenol. As far as we know, that's it?" Jerry nodded yes.

"Okay, it's only Tylenol. What specific question do you need to ask?"

"I'm not sure what you're getting at, Dr. Martin."

I turned to the other intern. "Deborah?"

"When did she take the pills?"

"EXACTLY. You need to know *when* she took the pills because treatment depends on that information *and* the blood level. What's the story, Jerry?"

"The blood Tylenol level was drawn about six hours after she took the pills."

"Okay. What would you do?" I addressed both interns.

Deborah spoke up first. "At that level I would definitely give acetylcysteine."

"Right. We gave it to her," I said. "Otherwise, what can happen?"

"Severe liver toxicity," replied Deborah. "The acetylcysteine prevents Tylenol from forming a toxic metabolite."

"Right." Clearly, of the two new interns, Deborah was the sharper one.

* * *

We went in to see Ms. McKnight. Not the most pleasant person, she so far had refused to talk to anyone. A tall, thin, flat-chested young woman, she sat up in bed with arms crossed and glared straight ahead. Based on a suicide note and the number of pills she took, her attempt was no gesture. She was angry because we saved her life.

"How do you feel?" I asked. She looked at me, then away, and did not answer. The cardiac monitor above her bed showed normal vital signs. By now her risk for liver toxicity was minimal because of the treatment she had received. As soon as she could be evaluated by psychiatry service, she would be transferred from MICU. I saw no point in spending more time in her room. We moved on to Room 6.

"Here we have the strangest case of all," said Dr. Clark. "Everyone, meet 'Jane Doe'".

"That's not her real name, is it?" asked Deborah.

"No. They found her in a parking lot. Comatose, no identification. She's been here since yesterday morning. I'm told she was intubated in front of a Cadillac. Anyway, she has severe aspiration pneumonia and is on the ventilator with one hundred percent oxygen. Right now, except for Mrs. Waldstein, she's our sickest patient. She's got a chance to make it. Nothing here that's irreversible."

"Jerry, did you call the police?"

"Yes, I called and asked if there is a Missing Persons report on someone of her description. A black woman about sixty years old. They haven't got back to me yet."

As we talked, the interns took notes. They seemed overwhelmed, but in less than two days they would know everyone in detail, including any new arrivals.

We stopped in Room 7 to see Mrs. Waldstein again. Her cardiac rhythm and blood pressure were holding steady. Arterial blood gases were adequate, albeit with artificial ventilation. She seemed in no immediate danger, so we moved on to Room 8.

"Last but not least, Room 8, Marie Jackson. Very sad case," said Dr. Clark. Before us lay an 80-year-old woman completely comatose and connected to a ventilator.

Jerry opened her chart and pointed to the top of one page. "What do you see there?" he asked the interns.

"A date."

"What's the date?"

"May third."

"Two months. She came to Mt. Sinai on May third for a dementia workup. Her private physician ordered all the right tests, but nobody ever asked her or her family about what to do if she needed resuscitation. Well, she went for a CAT scan of her brain, and guess what happened?"

"She arrested?" asked one of the interns.

"Right on the table. It was a mess, trying to get her intubated. To make a long story short, she must have been apneic for a good five to ten minutes.

After her cardiac arrest, which was on May sixth, she developed every complication. Pneumonia, kidney failure, sepsis. We've treated everything. Family won't let go. Neurology agrees she has severe hypoxic encephalopathy, with almost zero chance for meaningful recovery. Actually, they said that on June 1st. Here we are a month later."

Ms. Jackson, tube in throat, life supported by machine, had her eyes open but demonstrated no awareness of us or her surroundings. She just stared past us. Periodically there was a twitching, writhing movement of her face and mouth, an indication of partially suppressed seizure activity.

"Why does she need a ventilator?" asked Deborah.

"Good question," I said. "A patient who has only some hypoxic brain damage doesn't usually require artificial ventilation. Unfortunately, her pneumonia was so severe that her lungs became permanently damaged. She probably also has some emphysema, from years of smoking. Anyway, we can't get her off the machine."

"What happens when you try to wean her?" Deborah asked.

"We tried once. She lasted a day and then developed respiratory distress. We gave her family the option of not connecting her back to the ventilator, but they couldn't agree. Some relatives said yes, some said no. Finally, guilt prevailed. They asked us to reconnect her. So, we are not even trying to wean her from the ventilator. She would probably arrest again and it would be a bad scene."

"There's also the problem that it happened in the hospital," Dr. Clark added.

"Yes," I said. "But the family's not talking lawsuit or anything. It's just that because it happened here everyone is skittish about pushing them to let her go. I'd love to get Mrs. Jackson out of MICU but the ward isn't ready for her just yet."

The interns shook their heads. It would take time to adjust to this reality of modern medicine. With all our machines, we sometimes do more harm than good.

"Well, let's go look at x-rays. Afterwards you can come back and get to know your patients in more detail."

We went to the x-ray viewing room across the hall from MICU. About ten minutes later the phone rang in the viewing room. One of the house officers answered and took a message from MICU, then relayed the information to the rest of us.

"The overdose is here."

Comment

In these stories, dialogue is presented pretty much as it is spoken on rounds. You are right to be offended if you ever hear patients referred to as a diagnosis or organ. Phrases like "this overdose," "that gallbladder," and "the heart," when referring to specific patients, are not condoned. Unfortunately, doctors and nurses are incorrigible users of jargon, and it is not an easy habit to break. Despite the way some doctors and nurses occasionally communicate with one another, in my career, they invariably spoke to patients and families in a manner that was most respectful.

– END –

2. Overdose

Judy Bilowitz was only twenty when she came to MICU, but this was not her first hospital admission. She was diagnosed as a "depressed personality" shortly after puberty. As a teenager, she spent two long periods in Weathergill Pavilion, the state's top psychiatric hospital. Judy came from a prosperous family and could afford the best care.

With the aid of expensive tutoring, Judy made it through a private girls' prep school, graduating at nineteen. Unlike most everyone else in her class she did not go to college or take time off for travel. Instead, she stayed home with her parents and fifteen-year-old brother, an out-going and mentally healthy high school sophomore.

Judy's father owned a scrap metal company, and her mother was on the board of several important charities. The parents' financial and social success only heightened the pain of Judy's illness; their older child simply held no promise. She had no interest in college and was too withdrawn to find and keep a job.

Judy also had little interest in boys, nor they in her. Though attractive physically—she had a slim, well-proportioned body, fair complexion and features that made for a pretty face, with straight brown hair—her inattention and blunted affect tended to repel the opposite sex. Boys unaware of her psychiatric illness usually considered her "screwed up" or "weird."

She was not a virgin. At fifteen, she became pregnant and had an abortion in her eighth week. She was in Weathergill at the time of conception and the offender was thought to be another patient. Tightened supervision during her second hospital stay, at age seventeen, prevented another sexual liaison. As far as her parents knew, Judy used no birth control.

To the outside world, Judy at twenty didn't seem to care much about anything. She was incapable of relating to others and had few identifiable interests. Despite every material advantage, there was little to occupy her time. She stared at TV much of the day, sometimes read or pretended to read (all her books were essentially picture books), and occasionally worked in the garden.

She had been under the care of three psychiatrists since puberty. Her current therapist was Dr. Erasmus Cohen, a medical school faculty member in his late thirties and, at the time of Judy's MICU admission, considered the ablest psychiatrist on Mt. Sinai's staff.

Dr. Cohen's assessment was that Judy suffered from "schizo-affective disorder associated with depression," a form of psychosis usually treated with medication. In Dr. Cohen's best clinical judgment, she stood to benefit from Triavil, a combination of the antidepressant *amitriptyline* (also marketed alone as Elavil) and the anti-anxiety drug *perphenazine* (marketed as Trilafon). Based on its chemistry—three rings of atoms—Elavil is a "tricylic" antidepressant, or "TCA."

Triavil comes in various dosages; the dose Dr. Cohen prescribed for Judy was 2-25, twice a day. Each 2-25 tablet contains two milligrams (mg) of perphenazine and twenty-five mg of Elavil. Judy's prescription began in late March, a little over three months before she ended up in MICU.

Judy faithfully took the Triavil and seemed to improve. She became more talkative, took trips with her parents, and joined a local gardening society. Because of the favorable response, Dr. Cohen renewed the drug monthly; her last prescription for sixty tablets was filled June 20.

On July 1 Judy didn't come to breakfast as usual. At about 8:30, the maid went to Judy's room and found her unconscious on the bed, the empty Triavil container beside her. There was no suicide note. From this information, it was deduced that she took about forty of the Triavil tablets.

* * *

Overdoses can be classified as intentional or accidental. Accidental overdose occurs when too much of a drug is taken by mistake; this happens mainly among children and the confused elderly.

People who intentionally overdose are usually suicidal, although occasionally an excess of drugs is taken "just to get some sleep" or "to cure my headache." Most of the overdose patients admitted to MICU are, like Judy Bilowitz, intentional and suicidal. Only about half leave behind a suicide note.

Would-be suicides may choose either prescription or over-the-counter drugs. OTC drugs such as aspirin and Tylenol are, of course, toxic in large doses and can be lethal. In the 1980s and 1990s, prescription drugs commonly overdosed, besides Triavil, included Elavil and other single-agent antidepressants, Valium and other anti-anxiety medications, lithium (used in manic states), Dilantin (seizures), theophylline (asthma), and Darvon (pain).

TCAs presented a much higher risk from overdose than the other medications, because the end result was more likely to be fatal. The widespread use and potential toxicity of TCAs, plus the nature of the patients, accounted for three sobering statistics in the 1980s and 1990s. An estimated 500,000 Americans overdosed on TCAs each year of those two decades. TCAs were the number one cause of fatal overdose. And, over seventy of people who succumbed from TCA overdose were pronounced dead *before* reaching the hospital.

It must be accepted that the risk of suicide exists in any severely depressed patient. If the treatment of choice for depression was bottled water, we would no doubt see patients suffering water intoxication. They would be bloated, but few, if any, would die. Instead, the treatment for many patients was a drug that is potentially lethal in large amounts.

The manufacturer's Product Information Guide to Elavil states:

> High doses may cause temporary confusion, disturbed concentration, or transient visual hallucinations. Overdosage may cause drowsiness; hypothermia; tachycardia and other arrhythmic abnormalities; congestive heart failure; dilated pupils; disorders of ocular motility; convulsions; severe hypotension; stupor; and coma.

* * *

Judy Bilowitz arrived at Mt. Sinai's emergency room July 1, 1995, 8:55 a.m., deeply comatose. While one physician took a history from the parents, others intubated her and began artificial ventilation. Her stomach was evacuated with a large bore nasogastric tube and then aspirated to remove any residual pill fragments. Activated charcoal, a drug absorbent, was put down the tube to bind any tablets not yet absorbed into the blood.

Based on her coma, which takes at least a couple of hours to manifest, the ER physicians placed her suicide attempt between 11 p.m. June 30 and 7 a.m. July 1.

It took the ER doctors about two hours to stabilize Judy and transfer her to MICU. I saw her for the first time as she was wheeled into Room 1. My first impression was that she fit the picture of a near-successful suicide-by-drug patient: comatose; pale skin without makeup; hair all frizzled; face distorted by two tubes, one in the mouth and the other in her nose. From the history to that point, and my visual inspection, I surmised Judy's overdose was no "gesture." She fully intended to end her life.

The clear plastic stomach tube, inserted through her left nostril, was now jet black from the charcoal absorbent. This tube would stay in place at least two days so she could receive additional charcoal every six hours. The endotracheal tube stuck out from the left side of her mouth and was secured with white adhesive tape that circled her head; it would remain until she could safely breathe on her own.

The physical exam, which I did with the intern Deborah Hafly, can be summarized as follows:

- Body temperature: 97.6 degrees.

- Pulse: 120/minute (increased)
- Blood pressure: 123/82 (normal)
- Respiratory rate: 16 (provided by ventilator)
- Head: no bruises or any sign of trauma
- Eyes: closed; no eye makeup; pupils dilated equally and reactive to light; retinal exam normal
- Ears: normal
- Neck: no stiffness; carotid pulses equal and strong
- Heart: normal, except for fast heart rate
- Abdomen: no tenderness or swelling
- Arms and legs: normal; no needle marks or scratches
- Genital area: bladder catheter (inserted in emergency room) draining clear yellow urine
- Nervous system: in deep coma; no response to her name but responsive to arm pinching by withdrawing her limb; tendon reflexes equal and hyperactive in all extremities. Eye reflexes and eye movements appropriate, indicating no structural brain damage

* * *

After our exam we checked results of tests obtained in the emergency room. Her EKG showed no arrhythmias but the "QRS" wave pattern, generated by the heart's conduction system, showed slight widening, a common finding in TCA overdose. We would watch this closely since further widening could signal impending cardiac arrest.

Her chest x-ray was clear, ruling out pulmonary complications such as aspiration pneumonia and pulmonary edema. An arterial blood gas drawn shortly after intubation showed adequate oxygen and carbon dioxide levels. Other blood tests showed no electrolyte imbalance or disease of the kidneys, liver, or pancreas. Her pregnancy test was negative.

"Well," I said to Dr. Hafly, "she looks stable for now. She'll need an arterial line, which the resident can help you with. We'll need to check her blood gases throughout the night. Our job is to support her ventilation and watch for cardiac or neurologic complications. She took about 40 tablets. That's enough Elavil to kill her."

"What about the other ingredient, the perphenazine?"

"I'm not so worried about that. Perphenazine's probably contributing to her coma, but it doesn't have the same lethal cardiac and neurologic effects as the tricyclics, at least not in the dose she ingested. By the way, is there an antidote for Elavil overdose?"

Dr. Hafly thought for a moment. "I don't know. I guess not, or she would have received it by now."

"Right. But if a patient develops life-threatening side effects, particularly cardiac, we sometimes use IV physostigmine. It blocks the stimulatory effects of the Elavil."

"Why don't we use it now? Her QRS is slightly widened."

"Physostigmine has its own side effects and can be dangerous. Besides, it's not an antidote, just another drug to block Elavil's nastier side effects. The EKG should improve as the drug leaves her body. After you put in the A-line, read the review on TCA overdose. A copy is at the nursing station."

I gave her the exact reference and went to the waiting area to meet Judy's parents.

* * *

Her parents impressed me as decent, hardworking people, upper middle class or perhaps even wealthy, but not at all pretentious. Of course, no one is pretentious when their child is hospitalized, but I have seen parents whose life style and ostentatious behavior seemed to explain their child's psychopathic behavior. I didn't feel that way about Judy's mother or father. As a parent myself, I felt sorry for them. Sorry that they had such a burden of a daughter, that they were denied the pleasure of watching her grow and mature normally and, far worse, that they might lose her to a fatal overdose. I tried to stay professional and show empathy at the same time.

"Right now, she's stable," I said. "She's listed as critical, but her blood pressure and heart are holding up, and all her vital organs are working except for her breathing. The machine will breathe for her until she comes out of coma."

"What are her chances, Doctor?" The questions came from Judy's mother.

"Well, I can't give a definite percentage, but I'd say they're better than 50-50. The fact that she reached the hospital alive is a good sign." As soon as I said these words, I realized how unartful they were. *Alive* as opposed to *dead?*

"What do you mean?" asked her mother.

"Most people who overdose on this type of drug don't make it to the hospital. But most of the patients who reach the intensive care unit survive the overdose."

"If she makes it will she be...will she be OK?" asked her father.

"You mean, will she have any major impairment?"

"Yes, that's my question."

"It's impossible to say now," I replied. "Her heart and kidneys are not damaged, and there is nothing to suggest brain damage so far. If she doesn't wake up within about forty-eight hours, we'll do a brain wave study and some other tests to check for brain damage. Right now, we can explain her coma by the overdose, so we just have to wait and see how she does."

Judy's parents looked at each other but said nothing. They had no further questions for the moment, so I returned to the ICU.

About an hour later Judy seized. The seizure started as a jerking movement of the left arm and within seconds progressed to involve her whole body. Her heart rate jumped to 160/minute and respirations became jerky.

The ventilator cannot properly deliver air when the patient bucks and seizes. The machine lets us know things are awry by sounding off a loud alarm: BZZZZZZZZZZ! Every attempt to push air into Judy's lungs met resistance from her jerking diaphragms. BZZZZZZ ZZZZZZZZZZ ZZZZ ZZZZZZ BZZZZZZZZZZZZ!

Other alarms went off. The heart monitor sounded a repetitive PING! PING! because Judy's heart rate was much too fast. Then the IV infusion pump went BEEP-BEEP-BEEP to signal fluid backing up in the tubing, a result of her spasms.

For about a minute there was cacophony and confusion in Room 1. BZZZZZZZZZZZZZZZZZZ! PING! PING! PING! BEEP-BEEP-BEEP. BZZZZZZZZZZZZZZZZZZ! PING! PING! PING! BEEP-BEEP-BEEP. BZZZZZZZZZZ! BZZZZZZZZZZ! Through it all, Judy's body jerked and shook in the manner typical of a grand mal seizure. The first things to take care of in any life-threatening situation are ABC: airway, breathing, circulation. I disconnected the ventilator from the endotracheal tube and manually pumped air into her lungs with an AMBU bag. Dr. Hafly listened to her lungs to check the results of my effort.

"I hear good air entry in both lungs."

"Blood pressure's holding at about one twelve over sixty-eight," added a nurse.

"Good," I replied. "Let's give her ten milligrams of Valium and one milligram of physostigmine. Give the Valium first. We've got to break the seizure." About one minute had passed since the seizure began.

"Valium is in."

Thirty seconds later Judy stopped seizing. Valium works that quickly. The only problem is that the drug is short acting. It doesn't prevent recurrence of seizures, so a long-acting drug like Dilantin has to be started.

"Let's load her up with Dilantin. Give her seven hundred milligrams over about thirty minutes." I looked up at the monitor and found that her heart was still beating fast at one sixty. "And give the physostigmine," I added.

19

With the seizure under control, I reconnected the endotracheal tube to the ventilator. Next, we checked an arterial blood gas and electro-cardiogram. The cardiac conduction complex was still slightly widened but not worse than before, and her heart rate was coming down, now 135/minute. Blood pressure and urine output were good, and there was no apparent organ damage. Her brain might have suffered damage from the seizure, but it was too early to tell, especially with all the Valium on board. With Dilantin infusing into her vein, there was nothing more to do, at least for the moment. I went to write some chart notes.

Thirty minutes later Judy seized again. Her second spasm was not as violent as the first one. We again bag-ventilated her manually and gave another 10 mg of IV Valium. This time her seizure stopped spontaneously, just as the Valium was being injected.

A and B—airway and breathing—were secure but now circulation was a problem. Her blood pressure fell from 118/68 before the seizure, to a life-threatening 80/40, and her heart rate zoomed up to 160/minute. Low blood pressure—hypotension—is an ominous sign in TCA overdose. It often precedes cardiac arrest. A critical moment.

"Let's infuse normal saline, wide open," I instructed the nurse. "And give two amps of bicarbonate. Also, another milligram of physostigmine."

Saline to expand her intravascular blood volume and raise the blood pressure. Bicarbonate to alkalinize her blood and decrease the amount of active TCA. Physostigmine to lower her fast heart rate. If these maneuvers didn't work, the next step would be 'pressors', drugs that have a direct effect on raising blood pressure. Unfortunately, pressors also raise the heart rate, and Judy's was already sky high.

It was now 1 p.m. Since arriving to MICU around 10 a.m., Judy had received, all intravenously:

> 2 mg physostigmine
> 1000 mg Dilantin
> 20 mg Valium
> 2 ampules of sodium bicarbonate
> 500 cc saline, with more running in rapidly

My mind was racing. What else to do? I couldn't think of anything. We continued with manual ventilation. The ventilator might make things worse, perhaps lower her blood pressure by forcing air in too quickly. I kept an eye on the overhead monitor, which gave a continuous readout of heart rate, cardiac rhythm, and blood pressure.

"What about dialysis?" Dr. Hafly asked. "Can it be used to remove TCAs?"

"No," I explained. "Dialysis does nothing to speed removal of Elavil. The drug is mostly bound to large protein molecules which aren't removed with dialysis. It just doesn't work for tricyclics. If she makes it through this crisis, we'll continue putting activated charcoal into her stomach. Otherwise, we just have to wait for her body to metabolize the drug—and try to keep her pressure up."

A nurse cut in. "Pressure's ninety over sixty, Dr. Martin. Heart rate one forty."

"Good. Deborah, please listen to her lungs again. All this fluid can throw her into pulmonary edema."

The intern leaned over and listened with her stethoscope. "Her lungs are still clear."

I looked at the monitor. Blood pressure 100/65. Heart rate 135. I relaxed a little. I wouldn't have to tell Judy's parents the worst news imaginable.

* * *

Over the next half hour, the threat of cardiac arrest diminished as Judy's pressure and heart rate stabilized. We reconnected the ventilator and checked another arterial blood gas. Oxygen and carbon dioxide levels were adequate, thanks in part to the oxygen-enriched air provided by the ventilator.

Continued coma and need for artificial ventilation meant she was still critical, and still needed one-on-one nursing care. Every hour, Judy's nurses charted blood pressure, pulse and cardiac rhythm, urine output, fluid intake, and the level of her coma. Every four to six hours they charted arterial blood gases, body temperature, a cardiac rhythm strip, list of medications delivered, and a detailed clinical assessment. Besides keeping meticulous records, the nurses administered drugs and fluids, turned and cleaned her, and changed her bed sheets at least once every eight hours. Judy's care exemplified one immutable fact: no matter how sophisticated the technology, a critically ill patient needs constant *human* attention. Patients like Judy live or die on nursing care. Doctors may direct the show, but nurses give the care, and Judy had the best.

* * *

Judy remained comatose for thirty-six hours. The evening of the second day, she showed the first signs of waking up. Only then did I feel confident she would survive the overdose. Seizures were under control, and her blood pressure was steady at 120/74. Her young heart had withstood a massive tricyclic overdose.

As the coma lifted, her brain's respiratory center also recovered. By the morning of July 3rd, she was breathing entirely on her own, so we removed the endotracheal tube. A few minutes later we removed the still-black nasogastric tube.

With both tubes, out Judy was on her way to full physical, if not mental, recovery. Neurologic exam showed no defects, and her heart rate was a healthy 86 beats/minute. Her affect was flat but that didn't concern us; it is the norm for patients awakening after a severe overdose. Because of possible delayed cardiac side effects, we planned to watch her in MICU until at least July 5th.

July 4th was a hospital holiday. We made rounds as usual but all non-emergency tests and procedures were put on hold until the next day. As if in recognition of the holiday, Judy was well behaved. She ate some soup and other liquids and made no demands on the staff. We pulled out the bladder catheter and got her out of bed. Her parents were in and out most of the day, obviously grateful for her survival, and also worried about what might come next.

On the morning of July 5, now that Judy was awake and could at least respond verbally, her psychiatrist Dr. Cohen re-entered the picture. He visited her bedside for about fifteen minutes, then recommended a transfer to the hospital's psychiatry ward after her discharge from MICU. There he would reassess her need for antidepressant medication.

"Is she still suicidal?" I asked, and immediately felt foolish over the question. Given her history, when would Judy Bilowitz *not* be suicidal?

"She doesn't want to talk about the overdose right now," Dr. Cohen said. "I spent most of the time talking about other aspects of her life. She's still pretty numb. I think she'll open up more on Psychiatry." We agreed she could be transferred the next day.

* * *

That afternoon, suddenly and without any threat or warning, Judy began screaming. I was in MICU at the time. My initial reaction was that she hurt herself; perhaps she fell out of bed or hit her head. We rushed to her room. She was in bed, eyes half closed, screaming a high pitched

AAAAYYYYYYYYYYYYYEEEEEEEEEEEEEEE!

It was a wail to wake the dead.

We found no evidence for any injury. I shook her and she quieted down momentarily. Then she looked at us—at me, the two nurses, and Dr. Hafly standing at the bedside—closed her eyes and turned away.

"GO AWAAAAAY!" she yelled. "LEAVE ME ALOOONNNNNNE!"

I was very concerned. "Judy, what's the matter. What's wrong?"

"Where's GREGORY?" she asked, in a tone as if to demand we release someone named Gregory.

"Who's Gregory?" I asked one of the nurses, assuming there was some history I had missed.

"Beats me," the nurse said. "I don't know."

Dr. Hafly didn't know either.

"Judy," I asked. "Who's Gregory? Is he your brother?"

"AAAAAAAYYYYYYYYYYYYYYYYYYYEEEEEEEEEEEEEEEEE EEE!"

"I don't think Gregory's her brother," said the nurse. "I met him, and his name is Jimmy. Should we give her something, Dr. Martin?"

"No. Her vital signs are stable. Let's just watch her so she doesn't hurt herself. I'll call Dr. Cohen."

I put in a call to his office, but he was unavailable. I told his answering service it was important and to have him call back as soon as possible. Judy was in no physical danger but we could not keep her in MICU like this. At the least, her wailing was disruptive. More important, it was probably a sign that she needed to go back on psychiatric medication.

One of the nurses tried to calm Judy, but it was no use. Judy wasn't seeking reassurance or a kind word. She didn't want anything except "Gregory," and it wasn't even clear that she wanted him—if Gregory was a real person.

Dr. Cohen finally called back about an hour later. I told him what had taken place.

"Gregory is a male nurse she knew at Weathergill," he explained. "She brings him up during times of extreme stress. He was a calming influence during her worst periods there. I imagine she realized for the first time that she's in a hospital and called to him for help. I agree she probably should be started back on medication. It would be best if she can be moved to Psychiatry. Are you ready to release her from MICU?"

I was and I wasn't. I wanted her to go but I also wanted to monitor her heart another night, and cardiac monitoring was not available on the psychiatry ward.

Dr. Cohen recommended we begin Haldol, a major tranquilizer, and that she be transferred to Psychiatry in the morning. I wrote the order: 1 mg Haldol intramuscularly every twelve hours.

Haldol worked and Judy calmed down. There was no more screaming and the following morning, July 6th, she was transferred to Psychiatry.

Follow-up

Triavil was re-started on the Psychiatry ward but at a higher dose: 4-25. Judy's psychosis improved once again on medication, and everyone was encouraged. Mrs. Bilowitz agreed to administer the medication at home and to keep the container locked away. Under this condition, Judy was released at the end of July.

At home, either her mother or the maid gave out the pill, twice a day, and watched Judy swallow it. Then the container was secured, a precaution taken to prevent another suicide attempt. There were of course other ways for someone in Judy's situation to attempt suicide.

The new dose worked well and Judy seemed to improve. She sometimes went shopping with her mother and on occasion took one-day trips with both parents. She even attended two meetings of the gardening society in the home of a family friend.

For most of August, Judy was watched like a fragile child but, as she improved, her parents' concern over another suicide attempt lessened. Dr. Cohen saw Judy during this period and did not find her overtly suicidal.

Judy's parents so desperately wanted her to live a normal life. As time passed, they more and more treated her like a responsible adult. There was even talk with Dr. Cohen of allowing Judy to self-administer the Triavil, though no decision had yet been made.

Judy must have been aware of this change in attitude. Was she just waiting and plotting another attempt? Or was her mind too disordered to make such plans? Whatever the thought processes in her head, one day in December of that same year, Judy somehow got hold of the almost-full Triavil, supposedly locked in a kitchen cabinet. How she did so we never learned. Her father was at work, her mother was out shopping, and the maid had the day off.

If Judy hesitated or pondered or fought the temptation to repeat what she had done six months earlier, we'll never know. We do know that sometime after her mother left the house, which was around 11 a.m., Judy found and opened the bottle, swallowed all the tablets, then threw the empty container in the trash and went to lie on her bed.

By mid-afternoon, when her mother returned home, Judy Bilowitz was dead.

– END –

3.   Call NASA!

Part 1

"You asked them WHAT?" My voice was raised in mock anger, to show the house staff on morning rounds that Dr. Howard Stine's question was unacceptable. Shortly after admitting an 88-year-old man with pneumonia, the intern had posed a certain question to the patient's son and daughter.

"I asked them," Dr. Stine repeated, 'Do you want us to do everything for your father?'"

"And what did they say?"

"They said yes."

"I see." I waited a few seconds for someone to offer comment. Dr. Stine was far from the first neophyte physician to ask such a silly question, and he surely wouldn't be the last. Instead of responding, everyone on rounds—two interns, a senior resident, two nurses—looked past me in the direction of the patient, Jack Smilovsky. We were standing outside his room, and sliding glass doors made him easily visible.

I knew what the house staff were thinking. *Well, it's probably not a good idea for Mr. Smilovsky to receive too much heroics, but if that's what his family wants, what are you going to do?*

"Barbara, what do you think of Howard's question?" Barbara Milo, the resident on the case, had rounded with me many times and knew my feeling about this recurring problem. Barbara is quick-witted and able to display the right amount of sarcasm when appropriate.

Turning to Howard, with her head cocked slightly toward the patient, Barbara went right to it. "Do they want him dialyzed if his kidneys fail? Do we intubate him if his brain slips between his vertebrae? Do we send him for a heart transplant if he doesn't respond to drugs? Do we give platelet transfusions if his bone marrow goes zippo? Do we—"

"Okay, Barbara, thank you." I looked toward Howard but spoke to everyone. "WE don't know everything that can be done. How can you ask a patient's family if *they* want everything done? Medical technology is endless, infinite!

"Soon we'll be sending patients into space, for God's sake, to treat them with zero gravity! Do the Smilovsky children want us to send their father into space? Did you ask them?" Everyone laughed. At least I had their attention.

Dr. Stine was buried by the laughter but he managed to speak up. "Dr. Martin, what should I have asked his family?"

"Not a zero-option question. With what you asked, either they could say 'yes', as they did or 'no, don't do everything.' But saying no puts them on an instant guilt trip. Maybe their understanding of 'don't do everything' is that we'd let him die for want of an aspirin or a bedpan. Who knows? You didn't give them any realistic options. It was like you came out and said: 'Okay, we've got your father. Does he live or die?' What *could* they say? Now that they've said yes, you've left Mr. Smilovsky open for mega technology. Maybe not the space shuttle—yet—but just about everything else. Look at him."

I slid the doors open and we went in and stood around his bed. It was a pathetic scene. Mr. Smilovsky looked his age plus another ten years: gaunt, wasted, emaciated, out of touch with what was happening. His eyes were half closed and sunken into their orbits. His open mouth showed only toothless gums and a tongue moving ceaselessly back and forth, without purpose. He might be suffering, but nothing in his eyes or hands or mouth communicated any feeling. This was not a human being so much as a heart and pair of lungs inside an ancient body. Mr. Smilovsky deserved antibiotics, a warm bed, and kindness. He did not deserve, because he would not benefit from, artificial life support.

At the start of rounds we learned that Mr. Smilovsky had been in Mt. Zion Nursing Home for four years, the last two completely bedridden and demented from longstanding Alzheimer's disease. When he developed fever and shortness of breath, he was sent to Mt. Sinai Hospital's emergency room. Lacking any clear directive about use of heroics, the ER doctors sent him directly to MICU, where questions about how far to go were, apparently, first asked.

Now, at the seeming behest of his children, neither of whom, to be sure, had demanded anything in particular, we were obligated to do anything and everything to keep him alive. The medical diagnoses were pneumonia, sepsis, and dementia. Treatment was with antibiotics, fluids, and nasogastric feeding.

Mr. Smilovsky's condition was tenuous. Any hour he might

'need' an artificial ventilator for respiratory failure. An hour after that, he might 'need' infusion of dopamine to support his blood pressure. Then he might "need" a pacemaker, kidney dialysis, and a host of other readily available medical technologies.

For the moment, however, his care looked reasonable; he had not yet entered the realm of high tech. I was ready to move on, but the other intern on rounds, Pier Simpson, asked: "Aren't we obligated to do what's necessary? I mean, isn't that why he's here?"

Blessed be the intern who bids me to continue. Professional life would be lonely without someone to *teach*.

"Pier, how many people die each year in this country?"

The intern shrugged.

"Well, how many people are *in* this country. You need to know this bit of trivia first." After a few seconds of silence from Pier I said, "Anybody?"

"About three hundred million," said Molly, one of the nurses."

"Right. Now how many people die each year, of all causes?"

"About a million?"

"No, actually it's about two million. Now, excluding those who die before they can get to a hospital, and children, and accident victims, let's say that about one million mostly elderly people die of chronic disease or end-stage illness or old age. Furthermore, let's say they all end up in hospitals like Mt. Sinai, and that they all get connected to life support machines just as they are about to die."

"Dr. Martin," Molly interrupted. "Shouldn't we discuss this outside his room?" Actually, it didn't matter to Mr. Smilovsky, I was sure of that. But our proximity to the patient bothered Molly, so I agreed to continue outside. We walked out and closed the sliding doors behind us.

"For the sake of argument," I continued, "let's say that life support therapy prolongs each patient's dying by an average of two weeks. They will all die soon anyway, because that's the premise, but we're going to interfere with nature a little by instituting artificial ventilation, intravenous pressors, and any other life support deemed medically necessary. Furthermore, this is all going to be done in intensive care units like ours. How much are we talking about?"

As soon as conversation on rounds turns to economics, everyone perks up and listens. It never fails. I now had their undivided attention.

"It depends on what each hospital bill is," said one of the interns.

"Right. Let's say two weeks of therapy before each patient surrenders to nature—that seems about the average length of time ventilators can keep them going. Remember, they are destined to die anyway. Now the basic room rate is a thousand a day. Added to that are charges for antibiotics, respiratory care services, tons of x-rays and other odds and ends, roughly twelve hundred a day above the basic room rate. Twenty-two hundred a day is the average hospital charge for a MICU ventilator patient. It's a lot more if the patient is dialyzed or gets a pacemaker or has any surgery. Anyway, at fourteen days for the typical terminal ventilator patient, we're talking about a little over thirty thousand dollars each, and that's not counting professional fees."

No one challenged my estimates. "Some patients will last longer than two weeks, others will go quicker no matter what you do, but thirty thousand is probably a nice, conservative figure. Now, what's thirty thousand times one million?" This being the era before cell phones, a pocket calculator was brought out.

"Thirty billion dollars," said Dr. Stine, in a manner that suggested awe and respect for the number. The others just raised their eyebrows in acknowledgment. I heard one nurse mutter "Wow."

"That's right. Thirty billion dollars. Not the national budget, but not a small amount either. And for what? To prolong dying two weeks? It seems ridiculous, doesn't it? Fortunately, those one million patients don't all end up in our ICU or anyone else's. Many die at home, or in the nursing home, or even in the hospital, in a quiet room with their family at bedside and no tubes or machines."

"But you would save some of those patients," said Dr. Simpson. "How can you decide ahead of time when it's inappropriate to be heroic?"

This intern is a jewel, I thought. He must round with me more often.

"That's right. Statistically some of them might *not* die. They might go on and *live* on the machines. Like Mrs. Jackson."

"Who is Mrs. Jackson?" asked Dr. Stine.

"Barbara, tell him."

Barbara turned to face the intern. "Mrs. Jackson is an eighty-year-old demented woman who has been here about six months. She was only in MICU for two of those months. Now she's up on Tower

North. We can't get her off the ventilator. And no nursing home will take her *and* her machine."

Neither of the interns, Howard Stine and Pier Simpson, made any comment.

"Look, the whole point," I continued, "is that doctors have to make decisions. Ideally, life and death decisions should be made with the input of the patient and family. Mrs. Jackson's family, as I recall, was never given an option about what to do. Now they're stuck, and we're stuck. And Mrs. Jackson's stuck. Ask her if she's happy. She doesn't even know what planet she's on. Should we have to spend thirty billion dollars to keep one elderly, otherwise dying patient artificially alive?"

There was no answer. It was time to change course.

"Pier, would you intubate Mr. Smilovsky if he were ninety-eight?"

"Well, it depends on the circumstances." A beautiful hedge. No answer at all.

"How about a hundred and eight?"

"Maybe." Now I had Dr. Simpson on the defensive, and losing ground.

"How about if he was one hundred and ten years old, and you had documented evidence of metastatic cancer to every major organ."

"No, of course not, Dr. Martin."

"So, you're willing to draw the line somewhere. But you feel uncomfortable about Mr. Smilovsky because he doesn't have widespread cancer. Only pneumonia and sepsis, theoretically treatable conditions. I understand that. At least you admit there is a line to draw."

Dr. Stine spoke up. "Dr. Martin, how would you have handled Mr. Smilovsky's family?"

"First of all, I wouldn't call it 'handling.' Explaining the situation is what you really want to do, in terms they can appreciate. I've never met relatives who want their mom or dad or sister or brother kept alive as a vegetable on a machine. Well, I take that back. We had one a few years ago, but the daughter had a few loose bolts, so that doesn't count. She could never understand the difference between near-brain-dead and sleeping. Sensible families *don't* want relatives kept alive on machines, with no hope of return to humanity. You have to discuss the situation in these terms.

"We should simply tell them the truth. 'Your father is eighty-eight. He's at life's end. Nothing we do will restore his mind or body to anything better than he was last week. The most we can hope to accomplish is a return to his former state, demented and bed-confined. If his breathing stops, we're legally obligated to use machines to keep him going, unless you tell us otherwise. We'd obviously like to know his own wishes, but that's not possible, so I'm afraid it's up to you.'

"You'll be amazed at how often they will say, 'No, Dad wouldn't want that. Do what you can to make him comfortable, but no life-support machines.' Or, they might ask you for more information: 'What are his chances of getting off the machine once he's connected? What do you recommend? What would you do if this was your father?' The point is, you've established a dialogue and given the family realistic options. You can easily take it from there. If you get a clear sense that heroics and artificial life support are not to be used, you can order 'Do Not Resuscitate'; then, at least, everyone knows how far to go or not to go. If he's made 'DNR' we don't end up with a social service disaster like Mrs. Jackson."

Fortunately, Mr. Smilovsky did not need artificial life support. He survived pneumonia and was sent back to his nursing home. But the man in the next room didn't fare as well.

Part 2

Mr. Mordecai Zigson was 82 when he came to our ICU. For Mr. Zigson everything *was* being done. By default. He received medicine's top technology not because he requested it, or because his family demanded it, but because there was no one to call a halt.

Mr. Z had no relatives anyone knew about, only a legal guardian. In the nursing home he was thoroughly demented, though not as bedridden as Mr. Smilovsky. He could sit and walk with assistance but had to be fed by nurses' aides.

Mr. Z was sent to Mt. Sinai Medical Center for impending kidney, heart and lung failure. About to die, in other words. His mind was too far gone to give insight into his own wishes for treatment. Having no family around—there were rumors of relatives in faraway places, but we never saw any and no one ever called—we had to rely on his legal guardian, an attorney long ago appointed by the court.

The attorney's knowledge of Mr. Z's medical condition was close to zero. He preferred it this way "in order to stay objective and not bias myself." To help preserve his own state of blissful ignorance, the attorney never visited Mr. Z in the hospital. When confronted over the phone, on the day of Mr. Z's admission, with the important questions—How far should we go? Can we make him DNR? What would Mr. Zigson want if he could tell us?—the attorney was non-committal: "Do what you have to do."

What did we have to do? Was it right to assault Mr. Z's body with tubes, needles, monitors, a ventilator, and other assorted devices? Was it right to take over the function of his heart, lungs, kidneys, pancreas, and stomach without his consent? Was it right to feed his gut with food that never touched his tongue and replenish his blood with scarce blood products? Was it right *not* to do these things?

The ethical questions were weighty, but the practical answer to all was simple: protect yourself against the threat of litigation. In the climate of the time—the 1990's, and there's no reason to think the situation is any different in the early twenty-first century—no one could legally fault you for trying to save his life, only for letting him die.

Having no one around to call a halt, physicians often find themselves giving care they feel is ethically, morally, or socially wrong. If we let Mr. Z die a natural death (God forbid!) and his estate came up for probate, some long-lost relative might come galloping out of the west to pursue an award commensurate with the charges: wrongful death, medical malpractice, mercy killing, *euthanasia*. To the lay reader, this may seem an irrational concern, but it's happened before. Yet if he had a third cousin—or legal guardian—willing to say "No, don't do this," and that decision was consistent with our own sense of medical propriety, we could have stopped.

Mr. Z had no one, so we practiced medicine by default. And the default mode was *everything*. No one caring for Mr. Z thought it proper to begin artificial ventilation when his breathing failed. Artificial ventilation was begun without hesitation. No one felt comfortable about starting hemodialysis when his kidneys failed. He was dialyzed. And no one felt good about giving blood transfusions when his gut began to ooze the vital fluid. He was transfused.

When we consulted a surgeon to advise about the intestinal bleeding, she decided not to operate, but not because it was inappropriate—the guardian would have given permission—but because we were finally able to stem the bleeding with more conservative measures. "Call me if the bleeding resumes," she noted on the chart. She *would* have operated had it been necessary.

And when Mr. Z's heart began acting in strange ways—here a beat, there a beat, and frequently no beats for many seconds—the cardiologist didn't hesitate to insert a pacemaker, "considering that everything possible is being done for this gentleman."

By day fourteen of Mr. Z's stay in MICU, the same day I chided Dr. Stine for his 'do everything' question to the Smilovsky family, Mr. Z was fully hooked up: a human form who had long since lost his humanity, artificially maintained by the best medicine had to offer.

Through his mouth entered a foot-long, semi-rigid plastic breathing tube. Three quarters of this tube lay in his throat and trachea; the other quarter dangled outside his face and was connected via a different type of plastic tubing to the ventilator. Twenty-two times a minute the machine went whoosh! (air in), swishhh (air out). Whoosh!-swishhh, whoosh!-swishhh....

Another machine monitored blood pressure continuously via a thin plastic catheter sitting in his radial artery. A larger catheter invaded one of his neck veins, and through this an infusion of dopamine helped maintain his blood pressure sufficient to perfuse kidneys and brain. A nasogastric feeding tube entered his nose and ended in the small intestine; liquid nutrients fed through this tube could sustain his metabolic needs forever.

A bladder catheter exiting his penis allowed urine to flow freely into a bag for easy collection. The latest and most expensive antibiotics went through another thin plastic catheter in his right forearm. A rectal tube helped funnel his diarrhea, a side effect of the antibiotics, into yet another plastic bag.

On rounds we discussed Mr. Z from head to toe, noting tubes, machines, drugs, diagnoses. I was satisfied that things were being handled correctly from a strictly medical perspective, and had very little to add. What more could one say? Everything was being done, practically every organ was supported by some drug or device. Altogether we counted seven tubes and catheters (tracheal, rectal, two intravenous, arterial, bladder, plus one for hemodialysis), three life support machines (ventilator, kidney dialysis, cardiac pacemaker), and ten different drugs, including the blood-pressure-supporting dopamine. Whatever the outcome, the house staff were on top of Mr. Z's care, and the training program was being served.

Or was it? Each device or drug we used for Mr. Z was a major advance in medical therapy. Each, in its own way, has done wonders for patients. You can find many articles showing how each therapy has improved survival by some significant percentage. For example, thousands of people can lead productive lives because of kidney dialysis, without which they would have died. Other thousands live a normal life made possible by a cardiac pacemaker.

But were all these therapies *in toto* appropriate for Mr. Z? What is known about using multiple life support devices in elderly, demented patients? Do they help? Does there not come a point of no benefit, when the second or third or fourth machine will add nothing but expense and patient suffering? My medical resident Molly called it. "Dr. Martin, why are we doing all this to Mr. Z?" she asked. Not *for*, but *to*.

"We're caught, Molly. We have no choice. No one is taking responsibility for decisions about Mr. Z. We are in a medical-legal conundrum."

The nurses and house staff looked at me as if *I* should be responsible, and I became a little defensive. "*I* didn't order hemodialysis. Dr. G. started it." Everyone knew this, of course; I was just pointing out the obvious.

"Look," I said, "Dr. G. doesn't want to go on record as withholding a life-saving therapy. We asked his opinion about what to do for the kidney failure. What else could he say? Dialyze! Ditto the cardiologist and everyone else. Individually, everyone is doing what's medically correct. But when you stand back and look at the big picture, that's when you see it's wrong. As a result, we're *all* responsible." There was a general nod of agreement to with my analysis.

One more teaching moment before moving on from Mr. Zigson. I pointed toward his monitor, with its erratic heart rhythm. "We're like physiologic voyeurs," I said. "We're charting an inevitable, natural process with our machines. He's dying and we're recording it all, down to the last electrolyte and heartbeat. It's absurd, but at least there's one consolation in all this. My second law of intensive care."

"Second law? What's your first law?" asked one of the interns.

"Don't you know?" I asked the group rhetorically, relishing in the fact they would not know something I make up only for these rounds. Occasionally, I like to kick around pseudo "laws," to make some sense out of what we do. If my lead-in sounds more like physics than the mere opinions of a lung doctor, I figure the house staff are more apt to listen and remember.

As expected, no one knew my "laws" of intensive care. "Okay, the first law: If it happens here it happens everywhere. This kind of futile care occurs all over the country, every day. So our situation with Mr. Z is far from unique, and we shouldn't beat ourselves up over it." While not on the same level as, say, the law of gravity, this statement is certainly a truism, one that helps to put our situation in perspective.

"Dr. Martin, what's the second law?"

My grand finale. "The second law is something to keep in mind as you contemplate what we're doing here."

I pause for effect, then speak. "Money not spent on dying patients will not go to feed hungry children."

* * *

The medical and moral travesty continued for another week. After that, the dopamine infusion no longer worked and Mr. Z's blood pressure bottomed out. There was nothing else all our machines and chemicals could do. Nature won.

Mr. Z's total hospital bill in 1995 came to $73,485, or in today's dollars, just over 120 thousand. This amount did not include professional fees.

– END –

4.   A Strange Pneumonia

One day in March 1985—the year is important—we received a transfer from another hospital: Reginald Herbert III, a 46-year-old oil company executive. He came to us from a non-teaching suburban hospital, with an undiagnosed and progressive lung infection. For two weeks, his doctors tried in vain to diagnose the cause of infection, finally concluding that he needed an open lung biopsy.

An "open" biopsy is a major operation, literally an opening up of the chest cavity to remove a piece of lung tissue. Mr. Herbert was transferred to our care mainly because Mt. Sinai Medical Center is better equipped for this procedure. He arrived on a Friday afternoon, in preparation for surgery the following Monday. On exam he was short of breath, breathing rapidly, and had a temperature of 102. He was "acutely ill" and could only talk with great effort because of respiratory distress. We obtained most of his medical history from the transfer records and Mrs. Herbert, a trim, fortyish woman who answered our questions but never went out of her way to volunteer more than was asked.

The facts were meager. Mr. Herbert had been well until three months before hospitalization, when he first noted onset of fatigue and a dry cough. Two seven-day courses of antibiotics, as an outpatient, did not change his symptoms.

Initially, his outpatient chest x-ray was read as normal, so pneumonia was not a tenable diagnosis. He soon became quite ill with high fever, sweats, and persistent dry cough. At that point he entered the suburban hospital where he underwent a battery of tests, including fiberoptic bronchoscopy. All results were non-diagnostic. His white blood cell count was elevated, and he had fever along with frequent coughing and an abnormal chest exam, so pneumonia now seemed a good bet. Sure enough, a few days prior to transfer, a shadow appeared on the chest x-ray and his physicians came to recommend the open lung biopsy.

Mr. Herbert's travel history fueled speculation of an exotic infection. As an oil company executive, he had traveled to many countries, mostly in South America. Mrs. Herbert said he had spent about half of the previous two years abroad, in blocks of six to eight weeks. She never went with him because they had two teenage kids in school.

Did he ever have pneumonia before? "No," she said. Did he become ill on any of his overseas trips? Nothing that she knew about. Had either she or her children experienced any febrile illnesses in the previous year? "No."

What an interesting case! Middle-aged executive with fever and pneumonia of uncommon cause. We ran through the "differential" of possible diagnoses, and why he might not have responded to empiric antibiotic therapy. By the time of transfer, Mr. Herbert had already received five different antibiotics, two as an outpatient and three more in the suburban hospital. Any common or typical infection should have been clobbered.

There was no evidence for the usual causes of pneumonia, such as Legionnaire's Disease, mycoplasma, streptococcus, staphylococcus, and hemophilus. The one other infection that always has to be considered, tuberculosis, seemed unlikely. Tests at the suburban hospital, both the skin test and a special bone marrow exam, were negative for TB infection.

There is a 'waste basket' category of 'viral' pneumonia, often diagnosed on assumption, by excluding everything else. Viral infections are often hard to positively diagnose. In the 1980s they typically required checking blood samples weeks apart, and the blood had to be sent to a special state lab. We were not ready to call this a viral pneumonia.

There are many other infections in the world alien to most American physicians: malaria, schistosomiasis, blastomycosis, aspergillosis, tularemia, filariasis. Could Mr. Herbert have one of these exotic illnesses? Very possibly.

We also considered non-infectious problems like cancer, lupus erythematosus, and rheumatoid disease, but these all seemed highly unlikely. Even *acquired immunodeficiency syndrome,* or AIDS, was considered, though there was no history of homosexuality or drug abuse, the only associated risk factors known at the time. Even so, an AIDS antibody test was sent out prior to his transfer.

Whatever Mr. Herbert's diagnosis, we agreed with the need for the open lung biopsy. It just might reveal an unusual and treatable infection. Perhaps one out of a thousand pneumonia patients have to go through this procedure to secure a diagnosis.

* * *

Mr. Herbert went rapidly downhill. By Sunday evening, two days after admission, his breathing was even more labored, he was a bit confused, and his blood oxygen tension was falling. All signs pointed to impending respiratory failure. We intubated him and began mechanical ventilation. Unless the lung biopsy showed a treatable pneumonia, his prognosis for survival seemed poor.

He went to surgery Monday morning in critical condition: ventilator-dependent, breathing 100 percent oxygen, and semi-comatose. Under general anesthesia, the surgeon quickly opened his chest and excised a small piece of left lung. One half of the biopsy specimen went into a bottle of formalin for fixation and staining; thin slices of this piece would be examined under the microscope. The other piece went into a bottle of saline, for culture of bacteria and fungi.

Twenty minutes after the biopsy Mr. Herbert's chest was closed, save for a drainage tube that is routinely left in place. He went to the recovery room and then, an hour later, came back to the MICU.

Sadly, the effects of the operation, added to his debilitated state, made it impossible for him to breathe without the ventilator. We could not remove the endotracheal tube until he improved, and improvement would require a treatable diagnosis.

* * *

On Tuesday morning we had the answer. Mr. Herbert was suffering from *pneumocystis carinii* pneumonia, called PCP, the commonest type of pneumonia in AIDS patients. Coincidentally, his AIDS antibody test returned from the lab the same day. It was positive.

The pieces fell rapidly into place. Our patient had PCP, a classic presentation for AIDS, but his physicians, myself included, were somewhat fooled by his social background and our own inexperience with the disease at the time. How could an upper-middle-class executive have AIDS? In 1985?

But he did. And that is why none of the antibiotics had helped Mr. Herbert. He had not received any drugs that attack *pneumocystis carinii*, which is a type of fungus. We immediately began the appropriate antibiotic for PCP, trimethoprim-sulfamethoxasole.

Because Mr. Herbert was in MICU, and I was available when the diagnosis became established, it fell on me to tell his wife. How to do it? There was no point in being coy or misleading, as that approach invariably backfires. I had told many patients and families terrible news, but never had a diagnosis of AIDS been that news.

I met Mrs. Herbert in the ICU on Tuesday afternoon, as she was coming out of her husband's room. She was alone.

"Could we talk for a minute?" I asked.

"Of course," she replied, and I escorted her to a small conference room next to the ICU, where we both sat in comfortable facing chairs. "We have the results of the biopsy," I said, matter-of-factly. She looked at me without responding, waiting for me to continue. I hesitated a brief moment. The truth wasn't so easy to report after all. "It looks like he has the type of infection seen in AIDS patients."

I expected some expression of disbelief, or denial, or even anger, but she only said, "I see." If Mrs. Herbert was surprised at the diagnosis, she didn't show it. This woman seemed like a rock.

She didn't ask any questions, so I continued. "Also, the blood test sent out last week has just come back. It is positive for antibody to the AIDS virus."

In a most *un*inquisitive tone she then asked, "I wonder how he got AIDS?"

I wondered with her. "Did he receive any blood transfusions in the last five years?" I asked. "The blood of AIDS carriers can infect otherwise healthy people."

"No, not to my knowledge," she replied.

"He didn't use any illicit drugs, did he?" I hoped she wasn't offended by this question.

"No, of course not," she said in a monotone, showing no offense but also no emotion. I thought it peculiar that she seemed so much more certain about drug abuse than about blood transfusions.

Suddenly it dawned on me. She *did* know how he got AIDS and she *wasn't* surprised at all. It now seemed awkward to ask the obvious question, so I let it pass. I was not prepared to ask about the extra-marital sex life of Reginald Herbert III, father of her two children. Whether she knew about it or not, was immaterial at this point.

I did ask her one other question. "Do you wish to be tested?"

"No, Doctor," she said, again without emotion. "I don't think so. It's not necessary."

* * *

Over the next several days Mr. Herbert continued to do poorly. He did not respond to the antibiotic for *pneumocystis*, probably because it was begun too late and his infection was too far advanced. He remained ventilator-dependent and in a coma.

Meanwhile, the Herberts' family physician, who had followed him from the beginning of the illness, learned more about their marital relationship. They had not had sex together for over a year. His lack of interest, and some pictures of men Mrs. Herbert found in his suitcase, made her strongly suspect homosexuality. She presumed that much of his homosexual activity took place abroad. She also told her family doctor what she told me, that she saw no need to be tested for the AIDS virus.

Mr. Herbert continued to deteriorate and died seven days after the lung operation, from sepsis and respiratory failure. Mrs. Herbert did not grant permission for an autopsy.

Comment

By the end of 1981, the year AIDS was first reported, there were 281 known cases in the United States. Two decades later, worldwide statistics showed over 20 million dead and many more millions infected. Since then, dramatic strides in treatment have cut the death toll sharply, at least in the U.S. In the U.S. new AIDS cases total about 38,500 yearly, and deaths from the disease about 7,000.

The type of pneumonia that killed Mr. Herbert, PCP, is now much less common compared to the 1980s and 1990s, because of "antiretroviral" drug treatment for AIDS. However, PCP is increased in patients receiving chemotherapy for cancer, and immunosuppressive drugs following organ transplantation. In these groups, the mortality from PCP remains high.

– END –

5. Asthma in the Last Trimester

About five percent of the population in industrialized countries suffers from asthma. An asthma condition can range from minimal symptoms, with little or no impact on daily activities, to severe and life-threatening disability. Asthma can develop at any age. I have often seen asthma develop *for the first time over age 60*, and in people with and without an allergic history.

In an asthma attack, smooth muscles lining the bronchial tubes, the airways of the lungs, contract or tighten. This contraction (also called bronchospasm) leads to narrowing of the airways. At the same time the bronchial walls become inflamed and secrete thick mucus into the airway, causing further narrowing. To gain some idea of what it feels like during a severe asthma attack, try breathing through a straw with your nose plugged. As you breathe, gradually pinch the middle of the straw until it closes about half way. Now jog in place.

In people with asthma a variety of stimuli can bring on an attack of bronchospasm, including allergic reactions, upper respiratory infection (including the common cold), exercise, climatic changes, tobacco smoke, and emotional distress. Whatever the precipitating event, the result is the same: obstruction to air flow, wheezing, and a feeling of air hunger.

In a desperate attempt to bring in more air the asthmatic recruits 'accessory' breathing muscles, mainly in the neck and shoulders, and breathes faster. At the height of an asthma attack patients look like they just ran a marathon race. Keep breathing through that pinched straw and you will, too.

By definition asthma is *reversible* airways obstruction. The bronchospasm and excess mucous usually abate with appropriate medication. The operative word is 'usually.' Sometimes asthmatics don't respond to treatment, or respond so slowly that their condition requires hospitalization. Fortunately, only a small percentage of asthmatics ever reach this stage.

* * *

Delores Buchanan was twenty-four when she came to the medical intensive care unit (MICU). Diagnosis: severe asthma, complicated by a thirty-six-week pregnancy.

As a child Delores suffered from hay fever but not asthma. She received allergy desensitization shots from age twelve to fifteen. At eighteen, just out of high school, she first developed symptoms meriting the label of asthma: some wheezing and shortness of breath on exercise. These symptoms were controlled with oral and inhaled medication, and over the next three years she never required hospitalization or emergency room treatment.

After a year of secretarial school she married and shortly afterwards became pregnant. There were no complications of her first pregnancy, and at age twenty, she delivered a healthy baby boy.

At twenty-one Delores suffered her first bad asthma attack. It started with a sinus infection. Nasal congestion progressed to mucus in her throat, cough, wheezing, dyspnea, more cough, more shortness of breath, and finally a trip to the doctor. Antibiotics and an asthma inhaler did not provide relief. Her shortness of breath progressed and she came to Mt. Sinai's emergency department. The severity of her symptoms mandated hospitalization for intravenous therapy, but she did not require intensive care. She gradually improved and was able to go home four days later, on a regimen of asthma inhalers and pills.

Her asthma remained quiescent for a while. At twenty-two, she became pregnant again and delivered a healthy girl. During this pregnancy, she had no significant asthma symptoms. While in the hospital, she asked for and received one or two extra inhalation treatments.

After discharge, Delores underwent another allergy evaluation. Skin tests showed allergic responses to nothing more specific than dust and common mold. Desensitization shots were not recommended. She continued regular visits to the allergy clinic and, over the next eighteen months, her asthma remained under control, with just intermittent use of inhalers.

In 1987, she developed a severe asthma attack a few days after a head cold and was again hospitalized on the regular ward. After four days' therapy with intravenous medication, she was discharged on a tapering course of prednisone. Prednisone is a corticosteroid and the most powerful anti-asthmatic medication. She continued to do well with outpatient therapy.

In the summer of 1988 Delores became pregnant for the third time. The first two trimesters were uneventful; she used an asthma inhaler as needed, about once every few days, and did not need prednisone. At thirty-four weeks gestation her asthma symptoms inexplicably worsened. She soon began inhaling asthma medication almost every day, until things got so bad her husband brought her to the hospital. Shortly after she arrived in the ER my beeper went off. I called down right away. The ER secretary connected me with the physician on duty.

"Dr. Martin, this is Dr. Michael Highland, in the emergency room. I believe you know a patient who's here now, Delores Buchanan?"

I had not seen her since the last hospital admission in 1987. "Yes, I remember her. She's a young woman with asthma. What's happening now?"

41

"She's thirty-four weeks pregnant, with one fairly severe asthma attack. I think she should be in MICU. She's working hard to breathe. We started her on SoluMedrol (an intravenous corticosteroid) and IV aminophylline (a bronchodilator)."

"Do you have a peak flow or blood gas?" I asked.

"Her peak flow is only about 110 [liters/minute]. Let's see, I have her blood gas right here. PO_2 is 72, PCO_2 38, pH 7.43. That's on room air." These results showed adequate oxygenation and ventilation, not a life-threatening situation. At least not yet. But then there was the fetus to worry about.

"Is her OB going to see her?"

"Yes. Dr. Senior's her obstetrician. His resident examined her and doesn't think she's in labor. They'll follow her in MICU. but they think she's too sick to go to the OB ward."

"Okay," I said. "Send her right up."

In women with a history of asthma, there is a rule about the condition during pregnancy. One third will improve, one third will have no significant change in symptoms, and one third will worsen. Unfortunately there is no way to predict which patient will take which course. Experience with an earlier pregnancy also doesn't predict what will happen.

There is also a simple rule for treating the pregnant asthmatic. Treat the mother and the baby will be taken care of. If you don't treat the mother fully, for fear of harming the fetus, it can actually suffer from distress and hypoxemia.

Certain drugs should not be used during pregnancy. They include: tetracycline, an antibiotic that stains fetal teeth; Coumadin, a blood thinner that crosses the placenta to enter the baby's blood; most newly-released drugs, since not much is known about teratogenic effects; and any drug that might cause uterine contractions. This proscription still leaves available virtually all asthma drugs, including corticosteroids, the most potent.

Mrs. Buchanan was put in MICU Room Five. After the nurses checked her weight and vital signs I went in and introduced myself.

She nodded hello, smiled, and tried to look comfortable, but rapid breathing and contraction of neck muscles with each breath showed some distress. Her face, full from pregnancy, displayed the fear and apprehension of severe asthma. Sweat covered her brow. Nostrils flared with each inspiration. Medication begun in the ER had helped a little but her respiratory rate remained fast, about thirty per minute. Also apparent were a distended belly poking up from beneath the bed sheet, legs swollen with edema fluid, and wheezing, audible at the bedside without a stethoscope. In situations like this you don't walk in and ask, "How are you?"

"Well," I said, "your asthma is beginning to respond to the medication. Just to be safe, we'll keep you here until your asthma improves, then you can have that baby of yours."

"Good . . . I'm looking forward . . . to that."

She could not speak more than a few words without pausing to catch her breath. I ordered a chest x-ray to make sure we didn't miss pneumonia or some other acute problem. A chest x-ray is safe, especially in the third trimester, but as an extra precaution the mother's abdominal area is routinely shielded with a lead apron.

We inserted a catheter in her radial artery for frequent blood gas monitoring. An hour after arrival to MICU her respirations were still labored, and arterial blood gases showed no major change. Not a bad sign, but not good either. Her chest x-ray was negative.

She received three basic asthma drugs: intravenous infusion of aminophylline and steroids, and inhaled albuterol via a nebulizer every three hours. She also received oxygen through a nasal cannula. A cardiac monitor displayed her heart rate and rhythm, and a separate fetal heart monitor recorded her baby's heart rate. Mother's heart rate: 130 per minute, baby's 160. Both acceptable.

* * *

Mrs. Buchanan's condition made me ruminate on severe asthma, and all the bad things that can happen, including the worst. Most people probably think, *Well, you're not expected to die from asthma,* which, compared to cancer or heart disease, is a fair assumption. After all, asthma is a reversible condition, there's good medication for it, and every general physician is familiar with the symptoms and therapy. Yet each year in this country several thousand people *do* die from asthma, approximately 4000 a year even now, in the twenty-first century.

Reasons for asthma deaths are varied. Over- and under-medication have both been blamed. Some patients are at fault for not seeking prompt medical attention. And, sadly, physicians are sometimes culpable for sending patients home from the office when they should be admitted to hospital. For about fifteen percent of patients there is no explanation. They come for therapy on time, they get treated appropriately, but they just don't respond.

At Mt. Sinai Hospital we saw about one death a year from pure asthma, and as I left our patient's room I thought back to our last one, the sad case of Johnny Morgan. He was young, poor, and unemployed. And he smoked. It was his additional misfortune to have bad asthma from the age of fifteen, asthma

43

which, by the age of twenty-one, had landed him in the hospital twelve times, four of them in intensive care.

The pity of Johnny Morgan's asthma is that each attack was probably preventable, or at least subject to rapid reversal as an outpatient, given proper treatment. Still, after a week of in-hospital treatment his lung function did return to normal or near normal. Then he would go home, smoke, catch a cold or develop bronchitis, and land back in the emergency room. Sixty-seven emergency room visits in six years, not counting the twelve that got him admitted to the hospital.

Johnny was given countless regimens of tapering steroids, numberless asthma inhalers, and hours of instruction on how and when to use the medication. He was admonished about smoking so often that "nicotine addiction" came to be included in his list of discharge diagnoses.

The outcome was foretold in Johnny's outpatient clinic record, which included as many stamps of "NO SHOW" as follow-up notes by his clinic doctor. Two or three consecutive NO SHOW entries were followed by a cryptic "Adm Hosp - See Hosp Chart" [Admit to hospital - see hospital chart].

In June, at age twenty-one, Johnny developed progressive bronchospasm. His ever-present asthma inhaler provided relief for a while but after several hours, perhaps longer, he began to feel that symptom of relentless suffocation that had brought him to our ER so often. A friend drove him to the hospital, about four miles distance on city streets. The ride over, as we learned later, was a nightmare for driver and patient. Johnny rapidly grew more distressed and his friend drove faster, running through red lights and stop signs, finally attracting a police car close to the hospital. Johnny's friend stopped in front of the emergency room, got out of the car and ran to the officer who had pulled up behind. "My friend's not breathing!"

The officer ran to the car, saw the slumped-over young man, and pulled him out of the car. The friend ran inside and yelled for help. In less than a minute a first class, battle-ready, A-1 trauma team was hard at work on Johnny, his body now spread out on the parking lot pavement.

The ER team got him defibrillated, intubated, infused, catheterized and medicated, but they couldn't get him ventilated. They were about two blocks too late. Johnny Morgan's lungs were beyond resuscitation and he died right there, some thirty steps from doors marked "Mt. Sinai Hospital Emergency Department."

Autopsy revealed no illicit drugs or alcohol in his body, just the stiffest, most plugged-up lungs we have ever seen. A pure asthma death.

Johnny Morgan was our last asthma death, and I was frankly concerned we were at risk for another one—Delores Buchanan.

* * *

Whether from stress of pregnancy or severity of the asthma attack, or both, Delores Buchanan did not improve. Her peak flow stayed low, only about thirty percent of predicted. Arterial PO_2 remained safe at 70 to 90 mm Hg, albeit with extra oxygen, but her PCO_2 showed an ominous climb upward, to the mid-40s. In an acute asthma attack, the higher the PCO_2, the greater the severity.

The most severe asthmatics—patients with profound respiratory failure who are in imminent danger of asphyxiating—end up intubated and connected to a breathing machine, *if* they get to the hospital in time. Delores was not yet at this stage, but she was also not moving in the right direction.

On hospital day two we doubled her steroid dose (treat the mother) and started an antibiotic, erythromycin. We continued monitoring both maternal and fetal heart rate. Mother: 120, baby: 162.

The obstetricians saw Mrs. Buchanan twice a day. Their notes were terse and not generally helpful: "Not in labor. Baby OK. Continue current management."

"The baby's fine," Dr. Senior told me 48 hours into Mrs. Buchanan's unremitting asthma attack. "If you get her over this attack, we'll let her go to term. Her due date is almost six weeks away. Just in case, I obtained permission for a C-section. How's she doing?"

"Not so great," I said. "The attack hasn't relented. What if she doesn't improve, or gets worse? When would you want to do a C-section?"

"It's hard to say. There's a risk at thirty-four weeks. Also, if she suffered any hypoxemia during intubation, it could be a real problem for the baby." He was right, of course. Surgery during a severe asthma attack can be a nightmare for mother and the unborn child. In addition, the baby would be born premature. Two strikes is no way to start out life.

By the afternoon of the third day our patient was clearly tiring out. Incessant dyspnea, muscle fatigue, and lack of sleep were taking their toll. Her peak flow was now consistently *below* 100 liters/minute and the PCO_2 level was almost 50! Blood oxygen was still adequate, but everything else pointed to one inescapable conclusion: Mrs. Buchanan's asthma attack would not relent until she was delivered of child. I called Dr. Senior and gave him my assessment.

"You could be right," he said. I knew I was right, but he'd have to make the final decision.

"I'll be over in a few minutes to see her," he said.

Mrs. Buchanan didn't wait. Five minutes later she became more fatigued and then suddenly *unarousable*. A 'stat' blood gas confirmed the worst; she was severely acidotic from a buildup of carbon dioxide. Treat the mother!

An anesthesiologist was called and within minutes Mrs. Buchanan was intubated and connected to a mechanical ventilator. We had to give some IV sedation to coordinate her breathing with the machine. It was that or risk losing the baby to maternal distress.

Minutes after the intubation, Dr. Senior arrived. He saw what had transpired and immediately focused his concern on the baby. "What happened to the fetal heart rate when she was intubated?" he asked.

"Here, Dr. Senior." One of the nurse's handed him a long paper strip, a continuous recording of the baby's heart rate. He scanned the strip from beginning to end. For about 30 seconds, just at the time of intubation, the baby's heart rate had fallen to 130 beats per minute, signifying some fetal distress. Now it was back up to 150. Sedation had apparently not caused any major problem.

Turning toward me, he said, "What do you think?"

"I think the baby's got to come out. We've given her everything and she's going nowhere. Her lungs are tighter than on the day of admission. She's in a state of respiratory failure. I think we got to her just in time with the ventilator. I recommend C-section if it's at all possible." I knew it was possible, I just wanted him to make the decision. I don't like to force the hand of any surgeon.

"It's possible, just risky."

I pointed to Mrs. Buchanan. "True. But this is riskier. Besides, shouldn't a C-section be safer now that we can control her breathing?"

"Sure, but the baby will be born premature and could suffer more distress," he offered. "Of course there's also the risk of leaving him in there. (At that point we didn't know the child's sex.) What's the mother's PO_2?"

"One twenty. That's on forty percent oxygen."

He thought for a few seconds, then announced. "We'll do it. You'll take her back afterwards?"

"No problem. She belongs in the ICU. You get to keep the baby."

We went out together to speak with Mr. Buchanan about the emergency C-section. A factory worker in his late twenties, he still had on his blue work clothes and steel-toed shoes. We explained the situation, the risks both ways, the worst that could happen if we did and didn't operate. He was in a state of bewilderment and left the decision in our hands, essentially reaffirming his earlier permission for the C-section.

Dr. Senior next placed a call to the head of neonatology, activating the hospital's protocol for high-risk delivery. An hour later Mrs. Buchanan left MICU en route to Labor and Delivery, a floor above MICU. Safe transport required a team of four people: two orderlies to handle the cart, a respiratory therapist to breathe her manually with an Ambu bag, and a nurse to watch the maternal and cardiac monitors.

Once in the delivery suite, Dr. Senior and the anesthesiologist became responsible for her care. I went along as an observer and to help in any way I could.

* * *

"This lady is tight," said Dr. Kazeem, the anesthesiologist. "She's requiring a lot of ventilator pressure." I. T. Kazeem, a short, balding man in his early fifties whom I have seldom seen dressed in anything but green surgical, has probably given more high-risk anesthetics than anyone in the city. Seeing him in L&D did a lot to ease my own anxiety. His comment was also a question. Were we doing everything possible for Mrs. Buchanan's asthma?

"I know, her asthma's bad," I said. "She's on maximal steroids, the works. The baby's got to come out before she'll improve."

Dr. Kazeem turned his attention to the surgeon. "How quick are you, Dr. Senior?" A gentle reminder that speed was of the essence.

"Can you give me ten minutes of good anesthesia?" Dr. Senior replied.

"I can if her blood pressure holds up. I'm going to give her 100 percent oxygen."

"The baby'll love it," responded Dr. Senior. "He's already high on aminophylline. Fetal heart rate?"

"One sixty and holding steady," replied a nurse.

"Scalpel," ordered the surgeon. "Retractors." With those in hand, he told a nurse, "Move the light a little bit down her abdomen. That's better. Hold it."

The dialogue sort of reminded me of a grade-B movie. Only it was authentic, the patient's life *was* in the balance, and our sweat under the hot ceiling lights was all too real.

"Mother's pressure is one hundred systolic," said Dr. Kazeem. "How're you doing with her belly?" The anesthesiologist sat behind Mrs. Buchanan's head and could not easily view the operation. I, on the other hand, could see both Dr. Kazeem and the operative field.

"I'm getting there," Dr. Senior replied. He was assisted by a third-year obstetrics resident and two scrub nurses. Between them, I could see the incision. A wide low swath above her pubic bone exposed the distended uterus. Next Dr. Senior had to cut the uterine muscle. Slice. Slice. So easy in skilled hands. My thought at the moment: Be careful, a baby's in there!

47

He cut some more and the muscle parted. Two hands disappeared into the cavernous sac. Ten seconds later the hands came out holding a pink baby — a girl. He cradled her in his left arm and used his right hand to suction her mouth.

"Whaaaaaaa! Whaaaaaaa!" A sweet sound in the delivery suite. Success. Dr. Senior handed her over to the neonatologist.

"How's the mother doing?" Dr. Senior asked, ever so calmly.

"Holding steady. Sew her up," said Dr. Kazeem, relieved that one of his two patients was free and clear. I shared the relief. We all did. Whatever happened to Mrs. Buchanan, her premature infant entered life with an excellent chance of survival.

"She weighs 2200 grams (4.8 lbs.). A little slow in reflexes," said the neonatologist. "Apgar is seven. I think she'll be all right. We'll keep her in NICU (neonatal intensive care unit) for a few days."

I walked over to view the crying infant. She looked fine to me, just a little small. I returned to the operating table and slipped my stethoscope under the drapes, to auscultate Mrs. Buchanan's mechanically-ventilated lungs. Still wheezing, still tight.

I left the operating room to tell Mr. Buchanan the good news. He asked when he could see his wife and their baby. "Soon," I said. "Your wife first has to wake up from anesthesia. And the baby has to go the neonatal unit, where you'll see her behind a glass wall."

He smiled, grabbed my right hand and said, "Thank you, Doc."

* * *

I was right about her asthma. Despite the pain of a hysterectomy incision, Mrs. Buchanan began to respond to our drugs. Rapidly. Within 36 hours we were able to remove the endotracheal tube and disconnect her from the ventilator. She still wheezed, and her asthma attack was far from over, but recovery was now just a matter of time.

Her first post-extubation words: "When can I see my baby?"

"Soon, very soon," I replied. "We can't bring her to the ICU because she might catch something. And you can't go to her until we're sure you're stable. We'll watch you a few more hours, then take you to her room."

Mother and baby were reunited that evening. And the baby now had a name, Abigale Clarissa Buchanan.

Breast feeding was out of the question, due to all the drugs on board, but with some help Mrs. Buchanan bottle-fed and changed a diaper. The next day we transferred her out of MICU, to the OB ward, where her asthma continued to improve. As for Abigale, despite some prematurity and low birth weight, she did fine and went home seven days after birth, in the arms of her mother.

Follow-up

Mrs. Buchanan decided to have no more children and underwent tubal ligation. Her asthma continued to be easily controlled with pills and inhaled medication. As for Abigale Buchanan, she grew normally through childhood and showed no signs of asthma.

6.   "We can't kill your mother!"

As an intensive care doctor, I've dealt with many ethical dilemmas, most involving decisions to start or stop artificial ventilation. One of the most difficult was that of Mrs. Virginia Tyson, an 80-year-old nursing home resident admitted to the medical intensive care unit (MICU) April 27, 1989.

A month earlier, she had fallen and fractured her right hip. She underwent a hip repair and returned to the nursing home, but had not walked since. Additional diagnoses were rheumatoid arthritis, emphysema, and cardiac disease. Dehydration, on top of her bed-confined state and chronic lung disease, led to acute respiratory failure. Shortly after arrival to MICU we had to place an endotracheal tube through her mouth and begin artificial ventilation.

The severity of her condition made it impossible to remove the tube and discontinue the machine ventilation. Although her acute medical problems were eventually corrected, she could not be disconnected from the ventilator. Each attempt led to severe shortness of breath. On May 4, she underwent a tracheostomy, a procedure that places a short plastic breathing tube through an opening in the neck, allowing the larger and more uncomfortable mouth tube to be removed.

With tracheostomy, a patient can eat while receiving artificial ventilation. The 'trach' tube is also much easier to care for than a mouth tube, and can remain in place indefinitely.

Mrs. Tyson's need for artificial ventilation did not improve after tracheostomy. She simply did not have the strength to sustain breathing without the machine.

Her closest family members were two daughters, one of whom lived in a nearby state and the other far away, in Seattle. The nearby daughter stayed in town and visited her mother daily, and was in phone contact with her sister.

Mrs. Tyson remained mentally alert. She could not talk with the tracheostomy but was able to communicate with a pad and pencil. SIT ME UP. IS MY DAUGHTER HERE? MY THROAT IS SORE.

Reflecting a trait I've noted among the elderly in MICU, Mrs. Tyson never asked about her disease or prognosis. "We're trying to get you off the breathing machine," we told her often. She always nodded in appreciation but didn't raise any questions. She also never objected to the care we gave her.

I met with the daughter almost daily. A thin, pleasant woman, she was quite understanding about her mother's lack of progress. She never challenged what we were doing, and only asked that "Mother be made comfortable." I felt no communication barrier between us, and also saw none between her and the MICU nurses.

Considering Mrs. Tyson's age, chronic illnesses, and ventilator-dependency, we raised the question of additional life support should other organs fail. Mrs. Tyson and her daughter requested no further life support or resuscitative measures, and a "Do Not Resuscitate" order was entered in her chart.

No other organs failed, and her lung condition did not improve. She remained stable, albeit ventilator-dependent. Our hospital allows for stable ventilator patients to go to a regular ward, so on May 9 we transferred Mrs. Tyson out of MICU.

At the request of Mrs. Tyson's internist, I continued to follow her on the ward, and made another attempt to wean her from the ventilator shortly after transfer. When this failed, I suggested social service look for a nursing home that would take ventilator-dependent patients. Mrs. Tyson's original nursing home could not accept her back with the ventilator.

No matter how routine ventilators become inside a hospital, they are not routine in other facilities. In 1989 only two nursing homes in our metropolitan area accepted ventilator-dependent patients, and they were both full. Still, we had no choice but to look for placement of Mrs. Tyson in a chronic care facility. She could not come off the machine without dying.

Attached to the machine, she could in theory live many more years, although a sudden event, such as pulmonary embolism (blood clot in the lungs), could also end her life quickly. Her DNR status meant we would not intervene if another bodily system failed, but it did not change the day-to-day care she needed and received. I felt sorry for Mrs. Tyson and her daughter, but there was nothing more we could do except continue medical care and attempt placement.

On May 15 I got a call from the resident caring for Mrs. Tyson. "Her other daughter is here and wants us to turn the ventilator off. She says her mother wants to die."

"I'll be right up."

In a few minutes I met this daughter, standing alone outside her mother's room. The older of the two children, she appeared to be in her late 40s, physically similar but more aristocratic in bearing than her sister. As to temperament they seemed totally different. The Seattle daughter had only arrived that day but wasted no time in getting down to business: "Dr. Martin, I want Mother disconnected from the ventilator."

"What? Your mother can't live off the ventilator."

"I know that. I know what I'm asking."

She had already learned about our failure to remove the ventilator. Calmly, I expressed amazement at her demand.

"Why all of a sudden?"

"Doctor, it's *not* all of a sudden. Mother has always expressed her wish to die instead of being connected to a machine."

"But I've cared for your mother for three weeks. Neither she nor your sister said anything about turning the machine off."

"Did you ever ask them?"

"No, it never came up. We made her DNR, that was your mother's wish. But you're asking something totally different. If your mother had refused artificial ventilation before we began, it could have been withheld. Mentally competent patients have every right to make such decisions. But neither your mother nor sister ever made that decision. What you're asking now doesn't make sense."

"I'm telling you what Mother wishes. My sister was just too timid to bring it up."

Wow, I thought. There's something strange going on here. What, I didn't know, but it got stranger.

"Let's go ask Mother now," she said. In disbelief, I followed her into Mrs. Tyson's room.

There was no introduction to the subject. Not even, "Mom, I brought the doctor in to discuss this matter." Instead, she simply asked: "Mother, do you want to die?"

Mrs. Tyson nodded yes. There was no emotion to the nod. Just a dutiful "yes."

"See," said her daughter. "Now will you disconnect the ventilator?"

It was time to be more forceful. I had a tough and determined woman on my hands. "Could I speak to you outside?" She agreed, and we left Mrs. Tyson's room.

"I'm sorry but I cannot disconnect the machine," I told her. "I respect your wishes and am not going to ignore your request. But I'm not the only one caring for your mother. This will have to be discussed with other physicians and the hospital's attorney. You have to understand, what you're asking has never been done before in this hospital. There is no way any single physician or nurse can just go in and disconnect a ventilator. We can't just walk in and kill your mother!"

"I'm *not* asking you to kill my mother. I'm only asking you to let her die a natural death."

"I know that's the way you see it. But you have to look at it from our perspective."

"When can you call these other physicians and the attorney? I want to get this resolved as soon as possible. Mother's suffered enough."

"How long will you be here this afternoon?" It was one o'clock.

"Doctor, I'll stay as long as necessary."

"Okay. I'll make some phone calls and see what I can arrange."

I called the chairman of our ethics committee (of which I am also a member) and explained the situation. He agreed to meet the next day at noon. I then called the hospital attorney and outlined my understanding of the legal issues. She also agreed to the meeting. The nurses, social worker, and medical house staff caring for Mrs. Tyson were also informed, and by three p.m. I had everything lined up. I returned to the ward. This time both daughters were there. Somewhat to my surprise, the younger daughter expressed total agreement with her Seattle sibling, but also admitted to being "not very good at verbalizing Mother's wishes." Verbalizing? She hadn't ever *suggested* what now seemed written in stone.

"Are you sure your mother wants to die?" I asked the younger sister.

"Oh, yes. Mother told me that many times. She's said that for years. She just never got a chance to say it here." Her tone was unsettling, almost accusatory. I was glad a meeting was arranged for the next day. Let others hear this.

"Now," challenged the lady from Washington state, "will you disconnect Mother from the machine?"

"I already told you that's impossible for me to do. I've spent the last two hours arranging a meeting for tomorrow, at noon. Our lawyer and the chairman of the ethics committee will be there. Is that time okay?"

"Yes. We'll bring our family lawyer."

* * *

The next morning, May 16, I came to see Mrs. Tyson on rounds and was immediately confronted by the head nurse.

"Dr. Martin, Mrs. Tyson's daughters were here last night. They were asking the night shift why Mrs. Tyson was being tortured and why she can't be disconnected from the ventilator. Mrs. Tyson even wrote a note asking to be disconnected. The nurses are really feeling stressed by their attitude. What are you going to do?"

I reminded her of the meeting and left it at that. Clearly, this issue had to be resolved quickly. I took some comfort in realizing that, having called the meeting, the decision was now out of my hands.

There were twelve people at the noon meeting, held in a library off the ward: nine from the hospital staff, plus Mrs. Tyson's daughters and their attorney. I adopted the role of moderator, to both provide medical background and make sure the daughters' wish was fairly presented. It was also important that everyone understand the background against which such an extraordinary request was being made.

After introductions, I briefly presented Mrs. Tyson's medical history, emphasizing that at no time did she or her younger daughter ask for the ventilator to be turned off. I explained how she was made DNR, and that this did not translate into disconnecting the ventilator in an awake patient under any circumstances.

I also explained how, because of emphysema and other medical problems, her lungs were damaged beyond repair and that I saw no prospect for her living without the ventilator. I offered my best medical judgment that without the machine she would die within 24 hours.

Then, looking at the older daughter, I commented, "We were all surprised when you showed up and asked to have her machine disconnected."

I was not asking for a response, but she volunteered one: "I'm truly sorry I didn't come earlier, but it was impossible. I am now here to see that Mother's wish is granted."

Looking toward the younger daughter, I remarked, "I understand you are in agreement with this request?"

"Not only am I in agreement, it's what Mother wants. It's what we want. It's what should be done!" What conviction. Where had she been the last three weeks?

The floor was open for discussion. The night nurse on the ward spoke first. "Mrs. Tyson wrote me this note last night." The note was passed around. I had not seen it before. The ethics chairman suggested I read it out loud.

PLEASE LET ME DIE. I DON'T WANT TO GO ON LIVING THIS WAY. VIRGINIA TYSON

"Was either daughter present when she wrote this note?" I asked.

"No," said the head nurse. "Both had left the hospital."

The older daughter spoke up. "Look, I know this must seem strange to all of you, but you people don't *know* my mother. She never wanted to live like this. Mr. Barnes, the family lawyer, has known Mom for forty years." She turned to the elderly gentleman, at least as old as Mrs. Tyson.

"That's true," he affirmed in a creaky and barely audible voice. "She told me many times not to let this happen."

I could only wonder: Why had none of this been made clear prior to admission?

The ethicist spoke up. "I'm Dr. Knowles. I was asked to come because I head the hospital's ethics committee. I don't know your mother and have not cared for her, but I'm a physician and have cared for many patients in similar circumstances, that is, elderly patients connected to a ventilator.

"I think I understand what you're asking. One problem I think we're all having, at least something that bothers me, is how this has developed. You are absolutely correct. The patient has a right to determine her destiny. The problem, from a purely ethical and moral perspective is, what is her real wish? I don't doubt for an instant your sincerity. It's just that I'm having trouble separating your mother's true desire from what she may be expressing out of guilt, perhaps for what her illness is doing to the two of you."

There! He said what we were all only wondering. Was Mrs. Tyson asking to die so as not to be a burden on her daughters, especially the older one, for whom the constraints of time, if not distance, seemed more of a problem than the younger daughter? Or were the sisters merely conveying what was truly their mother's wish from the very beginning?

Mr. Barnes objected. "That's not true. Mrs. Tyson has always said she didn't want to live like this."

Dr. Knowles responded. "I don't doubt that, Mr. Barnes. And I'm truly respectful of the awful situation she's in. I doubt any of us would want to live under these circumstances. I'm just expressing why we're all so surprised, and why it's difficult to accept what you are asking. If she had made this wish clear from day one, and the family agreed, then I think ethically there would be less confusion on the issue. I'm not saying we'd take her off the machine even then. It's just that, from an ethical viewpoint, the request would seem less unreasonable."

"Are you saying you won't take my mother off the machine?" asked the older daughter, with a fair amount of indignation.

Good, I thought; let everyone see what I've been up against.

It was our lawyer's turn to speak. A former RN, she was compassionate and direct. "First, let me say that I understand your request. I really do. I know your mother has no chance of surviving off the ventilator, and I accept that it may be her wish to die rather than go on living this way. The truth is, under state law, we can't disconnect the ventilator. Your mother is awake and alert, and we can't do anything that will lead directly to her death."

"You mean I'll need a court order to stop the machine?" asked the older sibling.

"Yes, I'm afraid so. I must warn you, though, that no court in this state has ever granted such a request on an awake patient. And if one did, we'd have to appeal it. Also, I don't think there's anyone in this room who would personally disconnect your mother's machine."

"Speaking for myself," I said, "as one of her physicians, I could not disconnect the machine and watch her die, court order or not. Would any of the nurses be able to do it?"

The three nurses in the room quickly shook their heads, and the discussion was over. Mrs. Tyson's daughters had presented their demand, entirely reasonable in their eyes, but unreasonable from a legal and ethical perspective. The daughters had lost the first round, but they were prepared for the outcome.

Without missing a beat, the older daughter said, "Then we'll take Mother home."

* * *

Over the next several days, prodigious arrangements were made to transfer Mrs. Tyson to the home of a local relative. We made it clear to the daughters she could not be released until assured she would receive adequate care. Sending ventilator-dependent patients home is not impossible, and we have done it before. However, it takes a lot of planning and some commitment on the part of the family.

The hospital's attorney felt that we could not block Mrs. Tyson's discharge unless we had evidence the daughters might harm her. We had no such evidence. In fact, both daughters were accepting of our decision not to disconnect the ventilator, coming as it did from such a powerful show of force and determination. They cooperated with all the people involved in the discharge, including respiratory therapists, visiting nurses, and Mrs. Tyson's social worker. Arrangements to send a ventilator patient home ordinarily take at least a week, and they did not try to rush us.

On the evening of May 21, four days after our meeting, Mrs. Tyson was found dead in bed. Her daughters had not been there for several hours and the previous nurse check, only an hour earlier, had found the patient weak but otherwise stable. Her death was deemed due to natural causes. No autopsy was performed.

– END –

7. The Yellow Man

Willie Duncan's body was a mess, the end result of a pint of whisky a day for God knows how many years. He was only thirty-eight but looked sixty.

When most people think of end-stage alcoholics, the visual image is probably one portrayed by Hollywood: a drunk stumbling down the street, or sleeping on a bar stool, or beating his wife, or abandoning her children for the bottle. The theater is also a source of vivid impressions—for example, the character of Eugene O'Neill's alcoholic mother in his autobiographical *Long Day's Journey Into Night*.

Stage or screen, the portrayal is usually focused on the alcoholic's *behavior*: out of control, irrational, or self-destructive. But what about the *body*? Has Hollywood ever presented for our entertainment the physical persona of the terminal alcoholic? Hardly, and with good reason.

Maybe you'll see a close-up of a face just before the drunk slips into alcoholic stupor: grizzly beard, red lips, bloodshot eyes. And perhaps you'll hear some well-rehearsed lines: "I don't care—BURP!—if you leave me— BURP!—Give me a drink—BURP!" ...fade away. Whether in drama or comedy, the camera does not dwell on the drunk's physical features.

Movies and television should not be faulted for glossing over the true clinical picture. In many cases it's too unpleasant, too *gory*.

You could go into any large urban hospital on any given day and find a patient like our Willie Duncan. He's yellow, head to toe; the eyeballs give it away. Normally white, Mr. Duncan's eyes were a deep, obvious yellow, the result of liver failure and accumulation of yellow-tinged bile.

End-stage alcoholics have arms and legs thinned by malnutrition. Examine the skin of the forearms and chest, and you'll likely see purple blotches, the result of fragile capillaries and easy bruising. Take the bed covers off and you may find a distended, tense belly, like that of a child with kwashiorkor—a severe of malnutrition seen in third-world countries. The physiology is the same—massive fluid buildup due to lack of protein. Protein holds water inside the blood vessels. Victims of kwashiorkor are starved for protein. In contrast, victims of alcoholism like Willie Duncan have a destroyed liver and so can no longer manufacture water-holding protein.

Looking up from the beach-ball belly, you will often find a chest covered with red "spiders," superficial blood vessels in a star burst pattern about an inch in diameter. Press the center of one spider vessel and it will blanch; let go and it will fill quickly with blood from the center outward. These abnormal vessel clusters are another sign of severe liver failure.

The mind of the typical yellow man will likely be slipping away. Our Willie Duncan was confused and disoriented. He did not know the day, the date, or the president. (In the 1990s, older confused patients often answered "Roosevelt" or "Eisenhower"). Even when you think the terminal alcoholic is lucid, he is not. Ask him to count back from a hundred by sevens: "100...93...86...79..." He cannot do it.

There's more. Search carefully and you'll discover the patient is likely bleeding internally. As the liver shrinks from the effects of alcohol, the veins inside the esophagus, which connects the mouth to the stomach, become engorged with blood. Normally, esophageal veins route their blood through the liver. The more the liver shrinks, the more these veins distend until, like a balloon continuously filled with air, they burst open and spill blood into the esophagus. The dark red blood is both vomited up and passed in the stool, where it appears as mahogany-colored diarrhea.

Even though we commonly encounter patients like Willie Duncan, we can't help but stare in amazement each time another yellow, bloated, bleeding patient comes to the hospital. It is a startling spectacle.

Our Willie Duncan was certainly forewarned. He was now in for his seventh hospital admission in as many years. Long before alcohol turned his liver into a rock-hard lump of scar tissue, he was told what to expect if he didn't stop drinking. During every hospitalization he was advised, cajoled, threatened: *stop drinking.*

In the early days Willie Duncan had a wife, a brother and sister. His relatives were told to get him to quit alcohol or he would die from liver failure. Eventually his wife left him (or him her, it isn't clear which). His brother was killed in a fight, leaving only a sister as immediate family. He had no children.

Nothing worked for Mr. Duncan. Like most terminal alcoholics, he was poor. He had once held a steady job as a cab driver but was now on welfare and living with his sister. There was certainly no money for an expensive alcohol treatment program, even if he was motivated to join one. His sister once persuaded him to enter Alcoholics Anonymous. He attended meetings only a few months before the bottle lured him away.

Willie Duncan's case reflected a sad fact: it is far easier to convince patients to go on a diet, to exercise, or quit smoking, than to stop drinking. Alcoholism is simply—all too often—an incurable condition. Except for a few specialized centers, most of which are expensive and closed to the uninsured, medical treatment is relegated to the *effects* of alcohol, not to the addiction itself.

In truth, Mr. Duncan's alcoholism was as untreatable as terminal cancer. He came to MICU to die. The method chosen by his body was exsanguination. He was admitted one day in June with massive gastrointestinal bleeding.

In MICU, we estimated that his engorged esophageal veins oozed blood at a rate of about 200 cc's an hour. Without some intervention, his body would be empty of blood in less than a day. Long before that point he would die of shock.

Everyone in MICU knew Mr. Duncan was terminally ill. But only thirty-eight years old! How could we let him just bleed out? Even if therapy appears futile, we had to try something. We tried everything.

First, we replaced his blood. In the first forty-eight hours he received eight units of blood and two units of fresh frozen plasma. Shortly after admission, during his first blood transfusion, a gastrointestinal (GI) specialist passed a flexible scope—a procedure called "endoscopy"—into his gut, to identify the sites of bleeding.

As expected, the GI specialist found bleeding esophageal veins. These veins were injected, through the endoscope, with a latex material. (In addition to engorged esophageal veins, alcoholics can also bleed from stomach and intestinal ulcers. Ulcer bleeding occurs from erosion into an *artery*. Esophageal bleeding is from a leaky or ruptured *vein*. The two causes of bleeding are treated differently.)

Endoscopic latex injection stops hemorrhage by changing the free-flowing venous blood into a harmless clot, but the technique works only about sixty percent of the time. Initially it seemed to work for our patient. Then, just five hours later, he vomited up about 100 cc's of dark red blood.

The next therapy tried was intravenous injection of "vasopressin," a potent vasoconstrictor medication; its goal is to 'constrict' or close down the bleeding veins. Vasopressin has long been used to control GI bleeding. For stomach and intestinal bleeding, the vasopressin must be infused directly into the bleeding artery. This intra-*arterial* infusion requires threading a long catheter through the thigh artery and then into the bleeding vessel itself, a highly invasive and specialized technique.

For bleeding *esophageal* veins, alone among causes of GI bleeding, vasopressin works just as well when infused through a peripheral arm vein. We began Mr. Duncan on 0.4 units of vasopressin per minute through an arm vein.

For the next twelve hours he was stable: no bleeding. Then he retched, leaned over the side of his bed and vomited up several hundred cc's of dark red blood.

The GI service was called to the ICU. What to do now? Surgery was not a viable option. No good operation exists for bleeding esophageal veins, and Mr. Duncan would likely not have survived surgery in any case. There seemed but one more thing to try: a Sengstaken-Blakemore tube. This three-foot long, hollow tube, named after the inventing surgeons, was introduced in the 1950s. Once the main form of treatment for massive esophageal bleeding, the S-B tube is now used only rarely and as a last resort, when latex injection and vasopressin infusion fail.

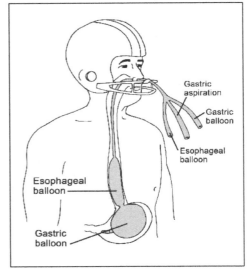

The S-B tube is affixed at one end with two inflatable balloons, one for the esophagus and a smaller balloon for the stomach (see drawing). When inflated with air, the esophageal balloon forces pressure against the hemorrhaging veins, much as you might stop bleeding from a cut by applying pressure. The esophageal balloon is basically a mechanical technique whose success depends greatly on proper positioning and the right amount of pressure.

To prevent the inflated balloons from moving and dislodging, the outside end of the S-B tube must be attached to a fixed object. Years ago, the outside part of the S-B tube was taped to the patient's forehead, but the tape always peeled off when the patient was moved. Then someone had a brilliant idea: use a football helmet. An S-B tube tied to the face mask of a football helmet works beautifully. If you see an ICU patient wearing a football helmet, you can bet he (or she) has esophageal bleeding.

An S-B tube was placed into Mr. Duncan's stomach and the balloons inflated. Amazingly, the bleeding stopped. But what a sight! A thin, emaciated, disoriented yellow man with giant belly, and wearing a football helmet emblazoned with the emblem of our city's professional team. For two days Willie Duncan lay like a wounded linebacker, the bleeding stemmed by fragile balloons pressed against his gut.

Light-hearted comments among the professional staff inevitably arise in this type of situation. They are 'insider' jokes, told to help relieve tension, to underscore the irony of what lies before us.

"Willie's trying out for the team. At the rate they're going, he'll make first string."

"I just got a call from [the Cleveland Browns head coach]. He wants to see Mr. Duncan right away. Let's clean him up."

"Willie should try out; he won't hurt their chances for the Superbowl."

That year, our pro football team and Willie Duncan were both losers.

***

Six different doctors became involved in his care this time around. If you asked each doctor what he or she honestly thought about his chances, none would admit to any optimism. I don't believe anyone held out much hope for Willie Duncan. I know I didn't, but still we tried. Was it inappropriate to do so? Should we have quit because our patient was an incorrigible alcoholic?

Given his age, I don't think so. You never want to let a patient's lifestyle influence your care. It would be ethically wrong to limit care *because* he was an alcoholic. Once you start making that type of judgment, you are on a very slippery slope. It is then only a small step to withholding care because someone smokes cigarettes, or eats too much, or doesn't get enough exercise, or drives a foreign car.

The only justification for holding back is if what you have to offer will not help the patient. It is as morally wrong to offer treatment that cannot benefit the patient as it is to withhold treatment that may. Not being a specialist in esophageal bleeding and liver failure, I was in no position to make any end-of-life decision about Willie Duncan. If the GI specialists wanted to try multiple latex injections and five S-B tubes (or surgery, for that matter), I could not legitimately object. Only physicians with knowledge and experience about the terminal disease should say there is nothing more to offer the afflicted patient.

Two days after the S-B tube was placed, Willie's vessels opened up. Dark red blood oozed out and around the S-B tube. Beneath his buttocks lay a puddle of mahogany-colored diarrheal stool. Before another unit of fresh blood could be infused, Willie's heart stopped beating. Willie Duncan bled to death.

Comment

We obtained permission for an autopsy from Mr. Duncan's sister. At autopsy his liver was markedly shrunken to only about half its normal size and weight, a condition known as end-stage cirrhosis. His esophageal veins were enormous, over two inches across. One vein had a large rent down the side, the site of his fatal bleed. There was no evidence for cancer or infection.

Chronic liver disease, including cirrhosis, is the ninth leading cause of death in the United States, claiming over 40,000 lives yearly. While there are many causes of liver failure, including infectious hepatitis, chronic alcoholism ranks as a major contributor.

Other life-threatening conditions related to alcohol include stomach ulcers, heart failure, vehicle accidents, and some brain conditions. Altogether, alcohol is directly implicated in 88,000 deaths per year in the U.S.

– END –

8. Adult Respiratory Distress

Joe Woodbury, 35 years old, was healthy until January 11, 1982, when he developed a scratchy sore throat, no different in character or intensity from what many of us suffer every year. Even in retrospect, those early symptoms suggested nothing more sinister than a minor upper respiratory infection. Two aspirin gave some relief, but that evening he also developed a slight cough, fever of 100 degrees, and a general achy feeling. His wife called their family physician, Dr. Levinson, who reviewed the symptoms over the phone. Everything certainly sounded like the classic flu syndrome, which usually gets better in three to seven days. Dr. Levinson reinforced the need for aspirin and asked to be called in two days if there was no improvement.

The next morning Mr. Woodbury was worse. He ached all over and cough was painful, so he went to see Dr. Levinson, who listened to his heart and lungs and heard nothing unusual. Eyes, ears, nose and throat were normal except for a flushing of the mucous membranes. On the outside chance that this was a bacterial infection, he prescribed an antibiotic, erythromycin, to be taken four times a day. He reassured Mr. Woodbury and asked him to call the next day if he was no better.

That evening Mr. Woodbury developed a mild sensation of shortness of breath, what physicians call dyspnea. Partly for this reason, he had a restless night and the next morning, January 13, was back in Dr. Levinson's office. Now there was also a new physical finding, cyanosis, a slight bluish skin color indicating insufficient oxygen in the blood. Dr. Levinson also found Mr. Woodbury's breathing heavier and deeper than normal. Everything pointed to a lung problem, so a chest x-ray was taken immediately. It was not normal. In the right lung was a grapefruit-sized, irregular white shadow just above the diaphragm, consistent with some type of pneumonia. Thirty minutes later Mr. Woodbury was admitted to the Medical Center's ICU (intensive care unit) with a presumed diagnosis of viral pneumonia.

The pace is fast in the ICU. Within the hour Mr. Woodbury gave a brief history to two doctors and a sputum sample to one of them, had a physical examination, several blood tests, and another chest x-ray, and began receiving intravenous fluids. One of the blood tests, known as arterial blood gas, showed his oxygen pressure dangerously low at 37 millimeters of mercury. Normal PO_2, as the test is abbreviated, is 85 to 100. To help counteract his hypoxia, an oxygen mask was set up to deliver 60% oxygen, almost triple the amount in room air.

I saw Mr. Woodbury soon after admission. His overall appearance can be described as "acutely ill," an observation based mainly on his dusky skin color, sweat over his brow, and obvious breathing difficulty. Also, his muscular build and full, round face made it certain he hadn't been ill for very long. Despite being short-winded, he was alert and cooperative. He also seemed strangely optimistic for someone so precipitously admitted to hospital, as if he perceived his condition to be easily curable by medical science. He had no particular reason to be cheerful, so I sensed this was his way of reassuring Mrs. Woodbury, who had just seen him and was now out in the waiting room.

I learned something of their family situation. The Woodburys had two children, ages four and seven. He worked as a foreman at the Ford Motor plant and his wife held a part-time secretarial job in the mornings while their younger child was in day care. Neither his children nor Mrs. Woodbury had been ill recently. Mr. Woodbury had not been hospitalized before, in fact had never been very sick, and did not smoke. He also had not been recently exposed to noxious fumes, chemicals, or dusts.

I went to see Mrs. Woodbury, a petite and pretty woman in her mid-thirties. She was scared, which considering the circumstances was an appropriate reaction. Before I could explain his problem, she wanted to know just how sick he was and "would he make it?" She might have sensed something in my demeanor, or my lack of smile, or the way I held my head.

Some ICU physicians believe in laying out all the worst possibilities from the very beginning, at least to the patient's family. This is called "hanging crepe," referring to the black fabric displayed at wakes or funerals. Once this approach is taken, anything bad that happens will have been expected; anything good will make the physician look like a hero. The truth is, I had seen many patients similar to Mr. Woodbury and "guarded" was an optimistic prognosis. Patients with such a rapidly progressive pneumonia can be dead a few days after their first symptoms. Still, except in the most obvious cases of brain anoxia, to emphasize only the worst possibilities is not fair to the family and could even be self-fulfilling.

I told Mrs. Woodbury that her husband had severe viral or bacterial pneumonia, and it was seriously interfering with oxygen delivery into his blood. His course appeared so rapid that if he did not begin to recover soon, he would need artificial ventilation and even that would provide only temporary support. We would order specific diagnostic tests, such as blood cultures and microscopic examination of his sputum, and continue treatment with oxygen and antibiotics. He would either respond or not, and we would know in 24 to 48 hours. There was a reasonable possibility he would improve but I could give no odds. She accepted this, which is to say all of her immediate questions were answered. I also called Dr. Levinson at his office and told him of the situation. He agreed with our approach.

The initial tests revealed increased numbers of infection-fighting white cells, both in his blood and sputum. We also found his sputum devoid of any bacteria, a finding that could be explained by his already brief use of erythromycin, which might have suppressed their growth. Alternatively, he could be infected with organisms that don't show up on routine sputum examination, including all viruses and some bacteria as well. In any case, the chest x-ray, white cell count and sputum exam all suggested a diagnosis of pneumonia, but did not reveal what specific type. Dozens of different organisms, including many species of virus, bacteria, fungi, and protozoa, could be responsible.

(By January 1982 AIDS had just been described and most physicians had never seen a case. Almost all the cases reported up to that time were from California or New York. Therefore, AIDS was never a consideration in Mr. Woodbury, although we did look for organisms now commonly associated with AIDS infections.)

We started Mr. Woodbury on two intravenous antibiotics, erythromycin and oxacillin. It was decided to continue the erythromycin because that is the best treatment for Legionnaires' disease, which we had not ruled out, and also for mycoplasma pneumonia. The bacteria responsible for mycoplasma pneumonia (*mycoplasma pneumoniae*) and Legionnaires' disease (*legionella pneumophila*) share certain characteristics: both are difficult to diagnose in the first few days of illness; neither can be seen under the microscope using conventional laboratory methods; infections caused by both usually respond to erythromycin. Thus, the drug seemed a logical choice for Mr. Woodbury. Oxacillin, a relative of penicillin, was chosen because it is excellent against staphylococcus. Staphylococci are a much more virulent group of bacteria than either *mycoplasma* or *legionella*; whenever a serious "staph" infection is suspected, treatment is begun immediately, without waiting for confirmation.

Mr. Woodbury did not respond. A few hours later he was still dyspneic and cyanotic, and his PO_2 was only 45. An oxygen pressure this low, especially while receiving extra oxygen, is life-threatening. Improving oxygenation at this point would require a major change in management, since the oxygen mask was ineffective. Mr. Woodbury needed artificial ventilation, which meant placing a tube in his trachea (the throat), a procedure called endotracheal intubation. We asked the anesthesiologist on call to come up to the ICU and intubate Mr. Woodbury.

Normal breathing, which involves inhaling and exhaling ten to sixteen times a minute, is silent, automatic and effortless. It is also not obvious to the observer. Mr. Woodbury was now breathing forty times a minute and working very hard at it. From across the room anyone could see his neck muscles rise and fall, a sure sign of increased work of breathing, yet each breath was ineffectual and their sum not enough to sustain life.

Despite severe respiratory distress he remained alert, so I carefully explained what was about to happen. I told him intubation was necessary, as the ventilator could not be effective otherwise. I explained he would have to be sedated for the procedure and that even when awake he would not be able to talk or eat. The ventilator would take over the breathing for him. He understood and asked me to call his wife, who had since gone home. I said I would call her afterwards. Fortunately, the intubation was quick and successful; he required ten milligrams of intravenous Valium for sedation.

The ventilator, a machine about the size of a dishwasher, was hooked up to his endotracheal tube via plastic hoses about two inches wide. The dials were set to deliver fourteen breaths per minute, with the volume of each breath quadruple the amount he was breathing on his own. To make it easier for him to tolerate the endotracheal tube and not "fight" the ventilator, we gave him another 10 milligrams of intravenous Valium.

A chest x-ray, taken with a portable machine, now showed an abnormal whitish haze in both lungs, consistent with some type of pneumonia. (The x-ray on the left is normal. The one on the right is typical of the severe pneumonia Mr. Woodbury had, showing the whitish shadows in both lungs.)

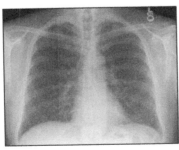 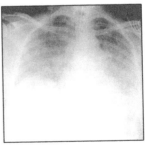

At this point the admitting diagnosis seemed correct: viral pneumonia. His sputum revealed no bacteria, and it was too early for culture reports to confirm any other diagnosis. But Mr. Woodbury's distress was due to more than just viral pneumonia. In just a few hours, once-healthy lung tissue had come apart, allowing plasma to leak out and flood spaces where only air should be. His chest x-ray showed the progression clearly. This flooding of the lungs—the medical term is "acute pulmonary edema"—is not what you see in the usual case of pneumonia. His condition had progressed beyond simple pulmonary infection.

* * *

Mr. Woodbury now displayed all the classic features of ARDS, the adult respiratory distress syndrome: acute onset of severe respiratory distress; bilateral "white-out" of the lungs as seen on the chest x-ray; life-threatening hypoxia. ARDS is one of those medical entities that has been around for a long time but only recognized and defined in the late 1960s.

ARDS was first characterized in a 1967 article published in *The Lancet*, England's famous medical journal, though the authors were all from the University of Colorado Medical Center. They described twelve patients admitted to the Rocky Mountain Regional ICU, all of whom had symptoms and clinical findings similar to each other and to our Mr. Woodbury: respiratory distress, severe hypoxia, leakage of fluid into both lungs, and a need for artificial ventilation. These symptoms in the twelve patients were precipitated by several different events, including viral pneumonia, pancreatitis and trauma to the chest or abdomen. A few of the patients were in shock prior to the onset of their respiratory distress. In fact, "shock lung" used to be another term for ARDS.

Five of the twelve patients died, a percentage that had remained about the same to the time when Mr. Woodbury was admitted. At autopsy, their lungs were a deep-reddish purple and much heavier and darker than normal, air-filled lungs. This reflected the tremendous inflammation and edema characteristic of ARDS.

ARDS was certainly not new in 1967. The type of patient with severe lung leakage has been described increasingly in the medical literature since World War I, when injured soldiers were often observed to die in fulminant respiratory failure. Autopsy studies in the 1930s and 1940s showed that many patients dying of shock had heavy, beefy lungs. In the 1950s and early 1960s, severe respiratory distress was described after such disparate conditions as open-heart surgery, compound leg fractures, and viral pneumonia. In 1966 the term "DaNang lung" was coined to describe the respiratory complications of soldiers critically wounded in Vietnam. In retrospect most—if not all—of these patients exemplified the adult respiratory distress syndrome.

The importance of the 1967 paper lay in recognizing a pattern of injury not unique to one cause but the final pathway for multiple causes, and in describing the clinical features of ARDS. This subsequently allowed many patients with ARDS to be diagnosed, studied, and treated in a rational, uniform fashion.

When all the causes are considered, ARDS turns out to be a common problem. In this country 190,600 cases occur annually, resulting in about 74,500 deaths (Medscape.com, October 2018).

Most ARDS patients are under the age of sixty-five, with no prior history of lung disease. ARDS is not due to heart failure, although a rapidly failing heart can sometimes cause a similar clinical picture.

ARDS is distinct from infant respiratory distress syndrome, also known as hyaline membrane disease, a condition that claimed the life of President and Mrs. Kennedy's son on August 9, 1963, two days after birth. Infant ARDS is due solely to premature birth and lack of a normal lung chemical called surfactant. While lack of surfactant plays a role in ARDS, it is not the primary cause.

Basically, ARDS involves the leakage of plasma and protein out of pulmonary capillaries, flooding millions of tiny airspaces. Why plasma and proteins leak out of the capillaries is not known. There are many theories, but none is universally or even widely accepted.

One problem in understanding ARDS is that most patients suffering the commonly-associated medical conditions, such as shock or viral pneumonia, do not end up with leaky lungs. It is unknown why some patients manifest florid pulmonary edema while others, in a similar clinical situation, maintain fluid-free lungs.

Though there have been some advances in the management of ARDS, none is considered specific therapy; in the jargon of intensive care they are referred to as "supportive," as opposed to "curative." One general advance is the ICU itself, a development dating from the 1930s when polio victims were first concentrated for better care.

The modern ICU, with electronic monitoring, artificial ventilators and specially trained staff, evolved in the 1960s and spread nationwide in the 1970s. Now, in the twenty-first century, every acute care hospital of more than minuscule size has at least one area where monitoring technology and skilled nursing are concentrated. This is the true meaning of intensive care.

Though the concept of the ICU makes a lot of sense intuitively, the benefit of ICUs in reducing mortality has not been proved for most illnesses, including ARDS. Given the critical condition of these patients and the fact that only about 40% survive the illness, it is not a study anyone cares to perform; no one wants to give any ARDS patient less care than that available in the modern ICU.

Another advance is the artificial ventilator, which has become more compact and reliable over the years. Unlike the old iron lungs, which hampered nursing contact with the patient's, today's artificial ventilators stand at the side of the bed and are connected to the patient through flexible tubing. They pump air into the lungs, rather than suck air from around the chest cage, which is what the iron lungs did. And modern ventilators can work round the clock for weeks with no more than routine bedside maintenance. It is seldom that any patient dies today from inability to be machine-ventilated.

Today's ventilators are also able, at the twist of a knob, to deliver positive end-expiratory pressure, known as "PEEP" (rhymes with beep). This extra airway pressure—maintained at the end of each breath—helps keep the alveoli open longer, so more oxygen can enter the blood. PEEP for ARDS was first reported in the 1967 *Lancet* paper, although its roots go back much further. In the late 1940s, pioneering jet aircraft pilots used positive-pressure face masks to increase their oxygen pressure at high altitudes.

Clinical use of PEEP was only conjecture until the Colorado physicians placed five of their ARDS patients on positive airway pressure. Three of the five lived whereas only two of the seven non-PEEPed patients survived. Because of the small numbers of patients, these results were, in the parlance of medical investigation, merely anecdotal, but they were enough to secure a place for PEEP in management. PEEP's main use is to increase oxygen pressure in the blood without using extremely high, and potentially toxic, concentrations of inhaled oxygen.

PEEP is not without hazards. Because of the increase in positive airway pressure, the lungs can sometimes "blow out" like a burst tire. PEEP can also prevent the normal flow of blood into and out of the heart, and cause heart failure. Those complications are manageable and to a large extent preventable with careful monitoring.

Machines that easily and rapidly measure blood oxygen and carbon dioxide levels (the "blood gases") are another evolutionary development. Various methods for blood gas measurement have been available for decades, but technically easy and rapid measurements only since the late 1950s, when new types of gas electrodes were introduced. Today, caring for critically-ill patients without blood gas measurements would seem like driving fast in a dense fog. You might make it but you would probably crash. Before the blood gas test was widely available, physicians literally guessed at the blood oxygen and carbon dioxide levels. It was a real crapshoot. Doctors now appreciate the unreliability, for sick patients, of trying to guess the levels.

Yet another advance has been a special type of cardiac catheter, a long, thin tube about 1/16-inch wide with a tiny, inflatable balloon on one end. The catheter is trademarked "Swan-Ganz" after H.J.C. Swan and William Ganz, two Los Angeles cardiologists. Drs. Swan and Ganz published their research in a 1970 issue of the *New England Journal of Medicine*, "Catheterization of the Heart in Many with use of a Flow-Directed Balloon-Tipped Catheter." For several decades after that, "Swan-Ganz" catheterization proliferated in ICUs. ICU staff spoke of inserting a "Swan-Ganz," "Swanning" the patient, or of the patient being "swanned." Like "Band-Aid", the brand name Swan-Ganz became a common-use noun. In later years, into the current century, the use of the catheter has tapered off, in favor of less invasive diagnostic methods.

The Swan-Ganz catheter modifies an old technique. Credit for the first cardiac catheterization is given to the German physician Werner Forssmann, whose story is now legend. In 1929, as a recently-graduated doctor working at Augusta-Viktoria Hospital in Eberswalde, near Berlin, Dr. Forssmann conceived the idea of threading a long, thin catheter through an arm vein and into one of the heart's right-sided chambers. His superior refused permission for such a daring study, so Dr. Forssmann clandestinely did it anyway, using himself as subject! He confirmed the catheter's placement with a chest x-ray and published the results in *Klinische Wochenschrift* later that year.

The medical possibilities lay dormant until the 1940s when Dickinson W. Richards, Jr., and Andre Cournand, working at Bellevue Hospital, began a systematic study of heart catheterization. Their work revolutionized cardiac diagnosis and paved the way for open heart surgery. In 1956, Drs. Forssmann, Richards and Cournand shared the Nobel Prize for Physiology or Medicine.

With or without the Swan-Ganz catheter, the key to treatment of ARDS is supporting the patient long enough for the lungs to heal. Once lungs fail in their capacity to deliver oxygen, either they must recover in a short time or the patient dies. Artificial ventilation for lung failure is measured in days or weeks, not months or years. There is no long-term "dialysis" as exists for kidney failure. If the patient is not destined to recover lung function, no amount of support can keep him alive indefinitely.

Patients who don't recover usually succumb to sepsis, cardiac arrhythmia, internal bleeding, or some other catastrophe. One of the saddest spectacles in medicine is to see a patient die with progressive respiratory failure despite the panoply of state-of-the-art, intensive-care technology. Those who do recover from ARDS, which is surely one of the most serious insults to afflict any organ, typically end up with some lung impairment, though they don't need supplemental oxygen.

* * *

With the ventilator Mr. Woodbury's PO_2 went up to 84 millimeters of mercury. This was adequate but far from normal, since he was inhaling 80 percent oxygen, almost four times the normal concentration. An expected PO_2 under these conditions is over 400. He was also receiving PEEP at 10 centimeters of water pressure, a moderate amount.

We gave him two grams of an intravenous corticosteroid, a powerful anti-inflammatory hormone often given empirically for ARDS in the early 1980s (today the drug is used much more sparingly in ARDS patients). Through a neck vein, we inserted a Swan-Ganz catheter and threaded it into his heart. Unfortunately, the catheter did not work at first, or rather the measurements did not make sense, as sometimes happens.

A chest x-ray revealed the problem. The catheter tip was coiled inside Mr. Woodbury's chest. After pulling back and reinserting the catheter, we were able to get the measurements needed to guide fluid therapy.

This was the scene about 7 p.m., some nine hours after Mr. Woodbury's admission. A young, previously healthy man lay semi-conscious in bed, sedated with Valium. In addition to the endotracheal tube, now firmly taped to his face so as not to slip out, four other tubes violated his body: the Swan-Ganz catheter, through a neck vein; an intravenous catheter, through an arm vein; a special arterial catheter, previously inserted into the radial artery in his right wrist and used for drawing blood gases and monitoring blood pressure; and a soft rubber bladder tube, earlier placed through his penis so that urine output could be measured.

Clear plastic tubing connected the several bags of intravenous fluid to Mr. Woodbury's body. In the aggregate, all the tubes looked like vines of some science-fiction forest. Interspersed between the vines were several pieces of electronic monitoring equipment: one to measure heart rate and rhythm, another to display the Swan-Ganz readings, and a third to show his blood pressure. Just to the right of his head was the ventilator with its reassuring "whoosh" of air being pumped into his lungs, a sound repeated fourteen times every minute.

At a glance, scenes like that surrounding Mr. Woodbury may appear unreal, certainly not the picture of human care. Doctors and nurses sometimes have to remind themselves that ICU patients like Mr. Woodbury are in fact human, possessing normal capacity to live and love. When we forget this, we are dealing not with patients as much as "heart-lung preparations," and the outcome is no more important than an interesting experiment. Intensive care can certainly give the appearance of an exercise in gross physiology. In truth, like some technologic fail-safe mechanism, internal reminders of the patient's humanity constantly arise and help guide us.

After discussing the next twelve hours' care with the nurses and resident staff, I left for the evening. Mr. Woodbury was one of five intensive care patients in our ICU at the time, yet by far the sickest. No major changes in therapy were planned, and we hoped for an uneventful night.

The next morning, January 14, Mr. Woodbury was not much better. During ICU rounds we reviewed the accumulated data: several chest x-rays, many blood test results, microbiology reports of his sputum, vital sign sheets. We double-checked the medication records and nursing reports. He was receiving the drugs on time and in the correct amount. Throughout the night he had been suctioned frequently, and turned in his bed as recommended. Laying in one place for prolonged periods is bad for any patient, especially those with ARDS.

Though Mr. Woodbury was receiving superb nursing and doctor care, he still showed no signs of improvement.

The information so far pointed to an infectious pneumonia as the initial event. Was he on the right antibiotics? The lack of definitive culture reports —still too early for many organisms to grow—and absence of bacteria in his sputum suggested a virus or one of the difficult-to-diagnose bacteria. Could he instead have an unusual fungal or parasitic infection, also difficult to uncover and requiring altogether different antibiotics? And if so, how did he get it? Mr. Woodbury had no history of a compromised immune system, the common setting for "opportunistic infections." They are called "opportunistic" because ordinary fungi and parasites take the opportunity to invade a weakened host. Unusual infections can also occur in bird-handlers, pigeon-breeders, and farmers, occupations remote from anything in his experience.

We decided to ask for help and called Dr. Dumont of the Infectious Disease Service. Since Dr. Dumont also ran the microbiology lab he already knew about Mr. Woodbury, at least about all his negative lab results. He sent his clinical fellow to the ICU and an hour later Dr. Dumont himself appeared, fully armed with all the data and his tentative conclusions. He didn't waste any time. "You've got to treat him for Legionnaires' and pneumocystis," he said.

We had continued the erythromycin because of possible Legionnaires' disease and had considered pneumocystis, but thought it a highly unlikely infection in Mr. Woodbury. Pneumocystis is a protozoan that occasionally invades kidney-transplant recipients and immunologically-compromised infants, but rarely healthy adults. Until Mr. Woodbury became suddenly ill, he was a healthy adult.

"I don't think it's pneumocystis but we can't be sure," he continued. "Let's stop the oxacillin and add Bactrim. If he doesn't respond in 48 hours, we'll consider an open-lung biopsy. Meantime, up his steroids to four grams a day and send a serum sample to the lab for fungal titers."

Bactrim, a trade name for trimethoprim-sulfamethoxasole, is the one of two major drugs for *pneumocystis carinii* pneumonia (the same pneumonia common in AIDS patients). Bactrim is effective and at the same time relatively free of major side effects. Since there was no reason not to follow his recommendations, we ordered the Bactrim and increased the steroid dose.

As for open-lung biopsy, this is major surgery and used for diagnosis only as a last resort. There was also no assurance that a piece of Mr. Woodbury's lung, under the microscope, would in fact yield an answer. He was not ready for an open-lung biopsy.

In the afternoon I met with Mrs. Woodbury. She came without the children, mainly because ICU policy does not permit children to visit. I told her about Dr. Dumont and our suppositions. She was not discouraged but also not encouraged. It was just too early to know which way her husband was headed.

Dr. Levinson also came by, and we discussed the case. He reassured me that nothing important was missed in Mr. Woodbury's past history and that whatever precipitated this crisis was acute and probably infectious.

Although private family physicians frequently will follow their patients in the ICU, it is not feasible to manage any critically ill patient from an outside office. It's no reflection on primary-care physicians, in this case Dr. Levinson, to have their ICU patients under the care of full time, hospital-based doctors. It is simply the best arrangement for the patient, a fact most office-based physicians well appreciate.

The rest of the day Mr. Woodbury maintained a PO_2 in the 60s on 10 centimeters of PEEP and 60% oxygen. On the evening of January 14, his second day in the hospital, his PO_2 suddenly dropped to 35; a portable chest x-ray showed that his endotracheal tube had slipped into his right lung, effectively bypassing his left lung which was now collapsed. The tube was pulled back, restoring breathing to both lungs and pushing the PO_2 back up to 59, still a low level but not life-threatening. A check of his electrocardiogram, urine output, and blood pressure uncovered no damage from the transient hypoxia.

On January 15 we received the preliminary culture, microbiology, and toxicology reports from specimens taken on admission. Everything so far was negative. There was no obvious or easily-diagnosed bacterial infection or toxin. This did not exclude the possibility of Legionnaires', *mycoplasma* or a viral infection, organisms which usually take weeks to diagnose because they require a convalescent blood specimen.

So, forty-eight hours after admission, we had no way of knowing what Mr. Woodbury had or if our treatment was effective. Whether or not he would improve seemed as likely to depend on the natural course of his illness as on any treatment. On Dr. Dumont's advice we continued the erythromycin and Bactrim. Throughout January 15 his temperature hovered between 101 and 102 degrees.

There was still no improvement on January 16. His PO_2 ranged between 50 and 60, on 60% oxygen and 10 centimeters of PEEP. His chest x-ray continued to display a "whiteout" in both lungs, and we continued to use small doses of Valium to sedate him and allow the machine to keep him alive. The steroids had not only caused his body to become puffy, a predictable side effect, but had also produced diabetes, a not uncommon result when massive doses are used; his blood sugar went to over 400 milligrams percent (normal is <100) and required insulin injections to control.

Now the picture was bleak, not because he was worse but because he was not improving. Patients who don't improve invariably die; ARDS is not a chronic condition anyone can live with. In desperation we began to consider an open-lung biopsy. What would a lung biopsy offer? Not much, unless he had some weird infection we had otherwise missed. What were the risks? General anesthesia and major surgery in a critically-ill patient. Perhaps an operative mortality rate of one or two percent. We discussed the procedure with his wife, with Dr. Dumont and, tentatively, with the thoracic surgeon. Somewhat reluctantly, since I doubted it would be revelatory, we scheduled a lung biopsy for January 18.

Mr. Woodbury showed the first sign of improvement on January 17. You wouldn't know it unless you had been following his blood gases. He certainly looked no different, and his x-ray still showed the diffuse haze in both lungs. But his PO_2 was now up to 95 on the same concentration of oxygen. This indicated some microscopic clearing of his lungs, not yet visible on the x-ray. In retrospect, this was a dramatic turnaround.

We lowered his oxygen a little and still his PO_2 held. On 50% oxygen, four hours later, his PO_2 was 92. We left things there. Something was working, probably the natural healing process we had been hoping for. We had no way of knowing whether the steroids or antibiotics or PEEP or all three had helped turn his course. As often happens in ARDS, there was no indication of why he was suddenly improving. We canceled the lung biopsy.

On January 18, breathing 40 percent oxygen, his PO_2 was 123. The pattern was now one of definite and sustained improvement. Except for the side effects of the steroids and the discomfort of the various tubes, Mr. Woodbury was doing well. We had stopped the sedatives and he was alert. His chest x-ray also began to show some clearing, the white areas melting away to reveal normal or clear lung fields. We removed the Swan-Ganz and arterial catheters and his urine tube.

As suddenly as he had deteriorated, he got better. Miraculously, we were able to disconnect the ventilator on the afternoon of January 18. The endotracheal tube was left in place another two hours, just in case he became worse, and he received humidified oxygen through the tube. There was no problem and he was able to breathe on his own, through the tube.

That afternoon the endotracheal tube was pulled out of his throat.

Follow-up

Mr. Woodbury was discharged from the ICU on January 20 and from the hospital on January 24. He returned to work February 15. I saw him as an outpatient the following week, at which time breathing tests, including an arterial blood gas, were near normal. Convalescent antibody titers were drawn. At a follow-up visit in June he was still doing well. Except for some slight decrease in exercise tolerance, he has suffered no noticeable aftereffects.

He didn't remember much of his ICU experience. He did remember going to the hospital and could recall the physical setting in the ICU, but most details, even from a patient's point of view, remained a blur.

We never made a specific diagnosis. All the antibody titers were non-diagnostic. In retrospect, considering all the negative laboratory results, a viral infection seems most likely, both for his early symptoms and the subsequent picture of ARDS. However, so many strains of virus can cause pneumonia that when only one person is infected, as opposed to an epidemic, like influenza, the responsible virus usually goes undetected.

Most viral illnesses are self-limiting, but sometimes they can progress and prove lethal. Fortunately, with the aid of intensive-care support, particularly artificial ventilation and round-the-clock care by nurses and doctors, Mr. Woodbury proceeded to get better on his own. Without this support he would surely have died.

– END –

9. Too Much Sugar, Too Little History

On morning rounds Peter Mance, one of the interns in MICU, presented a thirty-year-old woman admitted the night before with diabetic coma and ketoacidosis. The patient had developed gastroenteritis two days earlier, and stopped taking her daily insulin injections.

Dr. Mance had stayed up most of the night with his dehydrated, acidotic patient, balancing her blood glucose and acid levels with the proper amount of insulin and intravenous fluids. Before the insulin era, she would probably not have survived hospitalization. Now modern medicine, and a conscientious intern, had changed her condition from critical to stable in less than twelve hours.

In diabetes, the body's normal supply of insulin is either absent or deficient. Without insulin, a hormone made by the pancreas, glucose cannot enter the cells and be used as energy. Lacking insulin, glucose accumulates "outside" the cells, in the blood. Depending on the severity of diabetes, the blood glucose level may range from normal to over ten times normal.

Ketoacidosis, the most extreme state of uncontrolled diabetes, results from a sudden and severe lack of insulin; glucose builds up rapidly in the blood, to dangerously high levels. To forestall starvation, the cells turn to abundant fat as an alternative fuel. Metabolism of fat, less efficient than that of glucose, causes a buildup of harmful acid products called ketoacids—hence the term diabetic ketoacidosis, or DKA. The hallmark of DKA is an excess of acids and glucose in the blood.

DKA patients are very dehydrated because the extra blood glucose spills into the urine along with a large amount of the body's water. Glucose, a type of sugar, is not normally present in urine. "Tasting the urine" was an early way to diagnose diabetes (*not* a test of modern medicine). The full name of the disease is from an early description in Latin that referred to the urine: diabetes (to pass through) mellitus (honeyed).

* * *

Dr. Mance's patient was a "textbook" case of DKA. Not every MICU patient has to have triple organ failure or present ungodly ethical dilemmas. This patient, at least, presented a straightforward problem amenable to therapy. She also provided an opportunity for me to teach some medical history.

We went in to see her, a pleasant thirty-one-year-old Puerto Rican woman named Carlita Gomez. Mrs. Gomez looked and acted normal, which in itself was remarkable. From just her appearance, you would not know how sick she was a day earlier.

"How do you feel?" I asked.

"Much better, doctor."

"What happened that you had to come to the hospital? Did you forget to take your insulin?"

"No. Two days ago I began vomiting and was sick to my stomach. I didn't eat, so I didn't take my insulin yesterday or the day before."

"Why didn't you come to the hospital right away, when this all started?"

"I thought it would get better, like a stomach virus or something. Yesterday I got much worse and came to the emergency room."

"What made you finally decide to come yesterday?"

"I felt very dizzy and sick. My boyfriend said I looked very bad and he brought me."

"Peter," I said, "can you describe what she looked like on admission?"

"I saw her about twenty minutes after she arrived to the emergency room," he said. "She was very somnolent. I had to arouse her to answer questions, but she couldn't give me any information except her name."

"Was she short of breath?"

"Well, she didn't look like an acute asthmatic or anything, but I did notice her breathing was rapid and deep."

Rapid and deep, the classic breathing pattern seen in DKA, is the body's attempt to balance the excess ketoacids by hyperventilation or "blowing them off." The other classic symptom, excessive urination, causes great thirst and water ingestion.

"Mrs. Gomez, were you very thirsty before you came to the hospital?"

"Yes, I must have drunk twenty glasses of water yesterday and the day before. I couldn't seem to get enough water."

"I bet you went to the bathroom a lot, too."

"Yes."

"Has this ever happened to you before, that you had to come to the hospital for your diabetes?"

"I once came to the emergency room with the flu, and they said my blood sugar was high, but I didn't have to stay in the hospital."

"How long have you had diabetes?"

"Since I was twenty-one."

"Have you taken insulin that long, for ten years?"

"Yes."

"Does anybody else in your family have diabetes?"

"My mother, but she just uses pills. She doesn't need insulin."

"Who's at home with you?"

"Just my two kids. I'm divorced."

"How old are they?"

"My boy is seven and my girl ten."

"Did you have any problems with the pregnancies?"

"No. They were both heavy babies, though. The doctors said that was because of my diabetes."

"Who's taking care of the children while you're in the hospital?"

"My mother."

"Do your kids have diabetes?"

"No, not as far as I know. They seem to be fine."

Further history revealed that Mrs. Gomez was a patient in our hospital's diabetes clinic, that she was compliant with her insulin therapy, and that she did not suffer from the potential ravages of the disease, such as kidney failure and vascular disease. She supported herself with income from the state's Aid to Dependent Children program and some help from her mother.

We attributed her exacerbation to non-specific gastroenteritis, an inflammation of the stomach and intestines probably caused by a virus. She stopped taking insulin because she couldn't eat, but this only accelerated the vicious cycle leading to high blood sugar and DKA.

I reviewed Dr. Mance's detailed charting of insulin dose and blood test results. In the emergency room, Mrs. Gomez's blood glucose was 948 milligrams%, over nine times the normal value of 80 to 100 milligrams%. Her bicarbonate level was only six, about a quarter normal and indicating severe acidosis (the lower the bicarbonate, the more acid is in the blood). Dr. Mance's chart showed both her glucose and bicarbonate levels were returning toward normal, a direct result of insulin and fluid therapy.

"Let's see. She's now receiving two units of insulin an hour, right?"

"Right," said Dr. Mance.

"And her blood glucose is down to two hundred forty and bicarbonate up to nineteen?"

"Yes, those are the latest values," he affirmed.

"Well, it looks like she's on her way to complete recovery. You've done a good job, Peter." Turning to Mrs. Gomez, I asked, "How's your stomach? Do you think you can eat now?"

"I feel much better," she said. "I think I'd like to eat something."

"Peter, let's start her on a soft diet and advance to regular food if she tolerates that."

I thanked Mrs. Gomez, and our team stepped outside her room to continue the discussion.

"We should be able to switch her to subcutaneous insulin later today. That's what she uses at home. We'll keep her in MICU until she's off the intravenous insulin."

"Okay."

I turned to address the medical student, Sarah Miles, a bright and energetic woman in her early twenties.

"A fairly typical case of DKA, don't you think, Sarah? Have you had a chance to read about her problem?"

"Yes. I read about it last night."

"Good. You worked her up with Dr. Mance, right?"

"Yes." Sarah was on call the night before and had stayed up to help manage Mrs. Gomez.

"What did you read?"

"I read that DKA patients typically present with hyperventilation and stupor, and that reversal is fairly rapid with treatment, which always consists of fluids and insulin."

"That's right. What did doctors do with these patients before insulin was available? Anybody know?"

There was no answer.

"Starvation," I said. "Doctors prescribed starvation diets to their diabetic patients. Unfortunately, without insulin, almost everyone with ketoacidosis died. How long has insulin been available? Did your book mention that bit of history, Sarah?"

"No, I didn't see that," she replied.

"Well, how old are you, if you don't mind my asking?"

"Twenty-four."

I did a quick calculation. "Was insulin around when you were born, in nineteen sixty-five?"

"I think so," she said, perhaps wondering what the question had to do with our patient.

"Well, was insulin around in nineteen *fifty-five*?"

Bill Sedgwick, the other intern on rounds, spoke up. "I think that's when insulin was introduced. Nineteen fifty-five." He spoke with assurance, as if he really knew the answer.

"Bill," I said in a congratulatory tone, "do you play Trivial Pursuit?"

"Sometimes," he said.

"Anybody disagree with Bill?" I asked. No one answered. Everyone seemed to agree 1955 was when insulin became available. If so, they were only off by three decades.

Ignorance about this seminal event in medicine wasn't their fault, if it could even be called a fault. "History of medicine" as a subject is almost never taught in American medical schools. Even the historical aspects of everyday diagnosis and therapy are usually omitted. One principal reason is that the teachers are themselves often ignorant or uninterested, and that's too bad.

Doctors interested in history know that it helps provide perspective and humility in daily practice. It teaches us that today's "correct" therapy may be viewed as wrong-headed nonsense by future generations, much as we view primitive therapies of the nineteenth century and earlier.

Knowledge of historical events can also be of practical importance. For example, anti-tuberculous drug therapy was only introduced in the late 1940s. Anyone who contracted TB before then could not possibly have received effective drug therapy, yet on more than one occasion I've been told on rounds, by some well-meaning medical resident, that a patient received "TB drugs" in the 1930's or early 1940's.

Another time a house officer related a patient's treatment for Legionnaires' disease to a year before the disease was first described (1976)! Even local history is important. A patient could not have had a CT scan before the machine was available (in our hospital, 1978), yet I have been presented with the verbal reports of such phantom scans.

Like any history, of course, the history of medicine is far more than dates. The pioneering work of Banting, Best, Macleod and Collip in insulin, of Koch in tuberculosis, of Pasteur in rabies, and of Enders and Salk in polio vaccine, cannot be taught by dates alone. The stories behind major medical breakthroughs are invariably full of scientific excitement and human drama. Many are well-told in popular books, such as Paul DeKruif's *Microbe Hunters*, Michael Bliss's *The Discovery of Insulin*, and James Watson's *The Double Helix*. Still, it would be helpful if young physicians knew a few important dates.

"Nineteen twenty-two," I said. "Insulin was introduced into clinical medicine in 1922."

"Oh well," said Bill Sedgwick, suggesting by his tone that it really didn't matter whether it was 1922 or 1955.

"The first patient to receive insulin was a thirteen-year-old diabetic boy named Leonard Thompson. In what city?" I asked. If they didn't know the date, they also would not know the location of this medical milestone, but I was having fun, and they didn't seem to mind.

"Boston," guessed Dr. Sedgwick.

"No."

"New York," said Sarah Miles.

"London?" offered one of the nurses, in a final desperate stab.

"No. Everyone give up?"

All did.

"Toronto. The Toronto General Hospital. January 11, 1922. And who received a Nobel Prize for the discovery of insulin?"

"Banting," said Dr. Sedgwick, who was still out to win the trivia prize.

"You're half right," I said. "Banting who?"

"That's his last name. I don't remember his first name."

"Did anybody else get the Nobel Prize for work on insulin?"

No answer.

"How about Best? Banting and Best, does that ring a bell?" The two names, of course, are forever linked with the discovery of insulin. Even many grade-school students have heard of Banting and Best.

"That's right," said Dr. Sedgwick. "Banting and Best. I remember now."

"Yes," said Dr. Mance. "I remember, too. Banting and Best, but I don't remember their first names or anything about them."

"Actually, they are names you probably heard before you entered medical school. Like Salk and Sabin. Probably because of the Nobel Prize, I bet. Salk and Sabin got the Nobel Prize for the polio vaccine, and Banting and Best got it for insulin. Right?"

There was general murmur of agreement.

"Does anyone disagree?" If my questions seemed obnoxious, no one complained. In any case I felt compelled to continue, especially since no one had disagreed with my purposely erroneous statement about Salk, Sabin, and Best.

"Well, for starters, Sabin and Salk did *not* win the Nobel Prize."

"No? Sure they did," said Dr. Sedgwick. "That can't be."

"Sure they *didn't*. They developed and introduced the polio vaccines but never got a Nobel Prize for their work. The prize was given for earlier work on culturing the polio virus in monkey kidney cells, work that was published in 1949. So, who got the prize for work on polio?"

Now they were baffled. I was asking a bit of trivia they must have missed in school. No one answered, so I continued.

"The Nobel Prize was awarded to three Americans, Drs. Enders, Robbins, and Weller, in 1954, before the polio vaccine was even released. They were the ones who developed a method to culture the polio virus. Without their work there would have been no vaccine."

"Really?" asked Dr. Sedgwick.

"Really. And it was in Boston, too."

"Are you sure Salk and Sabin never got the Nobel Prize?" asked Dr. Sedgwick, still unbelieving.

"I'm sure. They got just about every other prize, but not the one from Stockholm.

"What about Banting and Best? Didn't they get it for discovering insulin?"

"Yes and no. That's an interesting story," I said. "Anybody want to hear it?"

I wasn't sure anyone did, but I wanted to tell it. It is one of the more fascinating stories of medical discovery.

"Yes," said one of the nurses. "Tell us."

"Right," agreed Dr. Mance.

Sensing a trace of sarcasm, I suddenly felt a need to defend the subject of medical history. Looking toward the patient I said, "There's more to a case like this than just glucose and bicarbonate levels. Sometimes we take these modern miracles too much for granted. Since you *insist*, I'll tell you about the discovery of insulin." And I did. For the reader, my conversation with the team that day is summarized in the next few paragraphs.

***

Before 1922 young diabetics were treated with low-carbohydrate, starvation diets. Even so, patients with DKA invariably died in coma. William Osler, in his 1892 *The Principles and Practice of Medicine*, a standard textbook of the era, wrote:

> In children the disease [diabetes] is rapidly progressive, and may prove fatal in a few days...as a general rule, the older the patient at the time of onset the slower the course...In true diabetes instances of cure are rare... Our injunctions today are those of Sydenham [an earlier physician]: `Let the patient eat food of easy digestion, such as veal, mutton, and the like, and abstain from all sorts of fruit and garden stuff.' The carbohydrates in the food should be reduced to a minimum.

Reflecting medical practice of the day, Osler's text devotes almost a full page to specific dietary recommendations, listing those items the diabetic may take and those that were prohibited. Among the latter was "ordinary bread of all sorts." Osler's comment on "medicinal treatment" of diabetes was an understatement:

"This is most unsatisfactory, and no one drug appears to have a directly curative influence."

In fact, no drug was even indirectly curative. On the subject of diabetic coma, Osler wrote:
"The *coma* is an almost hopeless complication."

Frederick Banting was a thirty-year-old surgeon from London, Ontario, who had the idea of isolating the specific secretion of the pancreas that lowers glucose in the blood. By the end of World War I, scientists knew some substance in the pancreas acted to lower glucose, but no one had been able to isolate it or use pancreatic extract successfully in diabetic patients. Banting moved to Toronto in 1921 to work in the lab of Dr. John Macleod, a Scottish physiologist who was an expert in the field of carbohydrate metabolism.

Banting was aided in his work by Charles Best, a 22-year-old medical student. The two of them succeeded in preparing an extract of pancreas that did lower blood sugar in dogs. This extract, of course, contained insulin. Under their direction, the first human trial of insulin took place in January 1922. (History records earlier animal trials of crude pancreatic extract, most notably by a Georg Ludwig Zuelzer in Berlin, but nothing came of that research.)

Leonard Thompson weighed only 64 pounds when he was admitted to Toronto General in December 1921. His diagnosis: diabetic ketoacidosis. He was initially given a diet consisting of only vegetables. Before he received insulin, Thompson's blood sugar ranged from 350 to 560 milligrams%.

Thompson was still in the hospital when Banting and Best were ready with their extract in January 1922, so he became the first human to receive it. According to the hospital record, Thompson's blood sugar fell from 470 to 320 milligrams% six hours after the injection.

It took Banting and Best two weeks to get more of the extract, and Thompson didn't receive his next injection until January 23. His blood sugar responded by falling each time. Thompson continued to receive insulin and was sent home on May 15, 1922, weighing 67 pounds.

From the very beginning, the discovery of insulin sparked controversy. Up until early 1922, Macleod had played no direct role in the discovery. Although he had acted as advisor on a number of the experiments, and Banting and Best used his lab, Macleod was actually out of the country in the summer of 1921, when most of the important dog experiments were accomplished.

The earliest scientific reports listed only Banting and Best as authors. In fact, Banting later wrote that he was discouraged in his work by Macleod, that Macleod told him "negative results would be of great physiological value." When it became clear that an important discovery had been made, Macleod got involved and orchestrated the production of insulin and further research into its use.

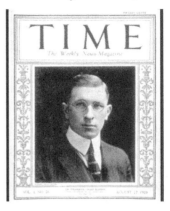

At the time, insulin was considered a cure for diabetes, so the discovery was quite a sensation. And no wonder. Patients near death were miraculously resurrected after only a few injections of the vital hormone. In August 1923, Banting became the first Canadian to make the cover of *Time* Magazine.

***

As expected, the discovery lead to the Nobel Prize for Physiology or Medicine. It was awarded in the fall of 1923 to Banting and . . . Macleod!

Upon hearing of the award, Banting was furious. In his view, Macleod had done none of the original work but only impeded his own brilliant research. Banting thought Charles Best should have shared the Nobel Prize.

Since Best was only a student at the time and did not present any of the research at meetings, as did Banting and Macleod, his role in the discovery

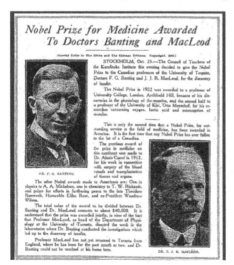

was not prominently featured. The Nobel committee was aware of Best—he was co-author on the original papers—but was more impressed by Macleod's senior status and the fact that he presented much of the research at scientific gatherings, one of which was attended by a Nobel committeeman. Also, by intention, the Nobel committee wanted to honor only two recipients (it was not until 1945 that three people would share a Nobel Prize in Physiology or Medicine). To the Nobel committee in Sweden, Banting and Macleod seemed the logical choices.

The total monetary award in 1922 was $24,000. Banting tried to correct the injustice by offering half of his award to Best. As it turns out, another scientist was also overlooked by the Nobel committee, a Toronto biochemist named J.D. Collip. Collip was responsible for purifying insulin far beyond what Banting and Best had achieved with their crude extract. In fact, Collip had purified all the injections given the Thompson boy except the first one. After being apprised of Banting's gesture, Macleod shared half of *his* prize money with Collip. Thus, the four men credited with discovery of insulin were Banting, MacLeod, Best, and Collip.

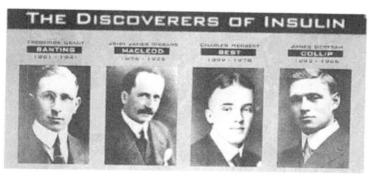

Even though their roles were publicly acknowledged shortly after the Nobel award, for the next two decades there was private, bitter feuding among all four men. They fought over priorities and who did what. Banting continued to believe that Macleod had hogged the limelight and deserved no credit for the discovery of insulin. Macleod thought Banting was an ungrateful young doctor who didn't appreciate how much he, the senior professor, had contributed to the discovery. Best, of course, was truly slighted by the Nobel Committee, and many contemporaries felt he should have been named a recipient of the Prize.

At least Best's contribution has been fully recognized by history, not to mention the University of Toronto. He outlived everyone in the story, dying in 1978 after a distinguished career as a professor of physiology. Collip also achieved long-lasting recognition for his pioneering work on purifying insulin. Macleod died in 1935, in Scotland. As for Banting, he died in a plane crash in Newfoundland in 1941.

* * *

"Well, that's enough about the discovery of insulin," I said. "Anybody have any questions?"

"What happened to the boy who got the insulin?" asked Dr. Sedgwick.

"Oh, glad you asked that. He lived another thirteen years, dying in 1935 at age twenty-seven, of severe bronchopneumonia. They did an autopsy and found the ravages of diabetes, including a shrunken pancreas. Any more questions?"

There were none.

"Okay," I said, "let's go see the next patient."

– END –

10. Crusade

Harlan Tembo has chronic bronchitis, a result of smoking cigarettes since he was 15. At age 57 Mr. Tembo was brought to Mt. Sinai Medical Center's emergency room one Monday in respiratory distress, blue, semi-conscious, and about to die. His diagnosis: exacerbation of bronchitis and acute respiratory failure. He was intubated, connected to a ventilator and sent up to MICU.

His hospital care reflected a quiet revolution in medicine. Before ventilators were available for patients like Mr. Tembo—that is, before the 1960's—he would probably have died. Now patients with acute and otherwise fatal lung failure are often saved by just a few days of 'ventilator support.' Even chronic patients with end-stage lung disease can benefit if their respiratory failure is acute and reversible. One of Mt. Sinai's chronic lung disease patients has been intubated at least nine times for acute respiratory failure. For Mr. Tembo, this was his first time intubated.

As late as 1967 there was debate about the utility of artificial ventilation in respiratory failure. Back then ventilators were much scarcer; now they are commonplace in every hospital. The only real debate over ventilator use today involves ethical issues, not medical ones.

After four days of artificial ventilation in MICU, Mr. Tembo could breathe on his own, unassisted by machine. It was time to begin my no-smoking crusade.

Every physician should mount a crusade when patients are most vulnerable, which is usually when they are ill and especially when hospitalized. It is not wrong to choose this time; it is wrong not to.

I am amazed how often physicians treat serious illness related to alcohol or tobacco, and do little (or nothing) to educate the patient. Why? Do doctors think patients automatically make the connection between habit and illness? In fact, patients all too often fail to make any connection unless directly and specifically told what it is.

Cynics may say I am wasting my time but evidence from various studies suggests otherwise. There is a positive influence on individual patients when *their* doctor gives advice in a forceful and direct manner. This is especially true about smoking.

The advice has to be more than mouthing a few words. The doctor (or nurse, for that matter) has to demonstrate genuine concern for the patient. Sometimes simple repetition will do it. Occasionally a threat works, as in:

"You'll need to find another doctor if you don't quit smoking."

But how do you communicate to someone you may never see again, or someone with only a grade school education, or someone who is a borderline psychotic? Sometimes reason, logic, and common sense are not enough. The message must always be personal and tailored to the patient's level of understanding. The important thing is to try.

* * *

"Let's extubate him," I said.

"Do you think he's ready?" asked one of the interns.

"Sure. He's awake, he's writing notes, he wants the tube out. Right Mr. Tembo?" He gave a vigorous nod. The nurse went to get the few items needed for extubation.

You know you can never smoke again, Mr. Tembo. We found cigarette smoke in your blood and that's why you ended up in intensive care." He nodded again, as if agreeing just so I would be sure to take the tube out of his throat.

"Once we get this tube out, if you go back to smoking the tube will have to go right back in. Do you understand?" He shook his head, meaning he wasn't going to smoke again.

The nurse returned with scissors and an oxygen face mask. I cut the tape securing the tube to his face, deflated the cuff inside his throat and pulled the tube out. Extubation is always a pleasure for patients, providing they are not gasping for air in the first place (as was Mr. Tembo on admission). If you can imagine a foot-long plastic tube stuck in your throat, making it impossible to speak or swallow or move your mouth, you can imagine the relief when it comes out.

"How do you feel, Mr. Tembo?"

"Better." His voice was hoarse but understandable.

"Do you know where you are?"

"In the hospital."

"When did you come in?"

"Last night."

"What day is it?"

"Tuesday?"

He had lost track of time, not uncommon in patients who receive artificial ventilation for more than a day.

"No. It's Thursday. You came in on Monday. You've been here for four days already. Do you know why?"

"No."

"Your lungs stopped working."

"Really? I guess I'm lucky to be here. Can I eat something?"

"Not right away. We'll let you have a little water, and then some soup." It's best not to give solid food right after a patient has just come off the ventilator.

"I'll be back later to talk to you about that cigarette smoke in your blood." Having finished our immediate task, we went to see the rest of our patients.

The next morning Mr. Tembo was like a new man. He had eaten his first regular meal and was well enough to leave MICU.

"Well," I said. "You're much better. You know you were quite sick a few days ago. A machine had to take over your breathing for four days."

"That's what they tell me."

"Do you know why?"

"Bronchitis, I guess."

"Well, that's true. You almost *died*. You came this close to being completely dead." I held up my forefinger and thumb an inch apart. "Do you know how you got that way?"

"No." He really didn't know or understand. But, sensing that the preacher was about to strike and remembering the conversation from the day before, he answered, "Cigarettes?"

"That's right, Mr. Tembo. You almost died from cigarettes. Your blood was filled up with cigarette smoke!" (Actually, his blood showed an excess of carbon monoxide, one of the toxic components of cigarette smoke).

"Well, I'm not going to smoke again."

I acted skeptical. "I've heard that before. Should we save this bed for you just in case?"

"Naw, you can give it to someone else. You won't see me back."

Time to stop badgering? Believe him? No. The physician has to make some *impression* on the patient, even to the point of looking silly or sounding obnoxious. Besides, I rationalized, I'm not only communicating with Mr. Tembo, I'm also teaching the house staff. Teaching them what? That they must do more than offer perfunctory advice about smoking.

"Mr. Tembo, I'm afraid your next cigarette could be your last." Then I delivered a non-sequitur: "Do you live near a funeral home?"

"Yes, why?"

"After you get home and decide to start smoking again, go to the funeral home before you light up. That way, if you die right away, they won't have to bring your body to the hospital." (Actually, this is not true. Even if you drop dead in the lobby of a morgue, the police will come and remove your body to the closest hospital to be pronounced. After someone pointed this out to me, I changed "funeral home" to "emergency room.")

"Well I'm not going to smoke again, you can bet on that."

"I hope not. But we'll keep a bed open just in case."

Mr. Tembo was discharged after a week in the hospital. He was admitted a year later for another exacerbation of chronic lung disease, but it was not as bad as the episode recounted above. He did not require intubation or care in MICU. And his blood carbon monoxide level was normal, so he had not resumed smoking.

"What made you quit?" I asked him.

"Well, Doctor Martin," he said, "I remember what you told me last year. So I just gave it up. And I don't miss it at all."

* * *

I don't know how many times I've taken cigarette packs from a patient's bed stand—always with their permission—or used my funeral home plea to get across my smoking-is-bad-for-you message. "What funeral home do you do business with?" "Is your will made out?"

I probably said something similar a hundred times over the years. Questions of this nature always got the attention of my addicted smokers, and if they made at least one quit the habit, it was worth the effort.

For Amanda Wiggins though, none of my usual messages got through. She had chronic lung disease and always complained of being "short winded." That was her constant complaint during one hospitalization on the medical ward. (She had been in the intensive care unit once before, but on this hospital stay she did not need the ICU. Also, note that this admission occurred before our hospital became a smoke-free institution.)

Neither fear of funeral homes nor emergency rooms nor ventilators nor lung cancer nor skin wrinkles made any dent in Mrs. Wiggins' smoking addiction. She was incorrigible. She continued to smoke in her hospital room and in the ward lounge even as we treated her for smoking-related chronic lung disease.

Psychiatrically Mrs. Wiggins was a "borderline" personality disorder— not psychotic, but with a tendency in that direction. Her anchor in life seemed to be the bible and fundamentalist religion. I saw this belief as a wedge to change her smoking behavior.

One day on the ward, as she complained about her shortness of breath, I auditioned my new message. I made sure her nurse was there; no one would probably believe me if Mrs. Wiggins really did quit smoking.

"Amanda, we can't get you better if you continue to smoke."

"I'll quit," she said, in a manner which conveyed just the opposite intention.

"You've got to quit."

"I'll quit. I want to get better."

"You're gonna die!"

"Don't say that, Dr. Martin. If I quit will I get better?"

"How are you going to quit? You've promised me a hundred times and you always go back to smoking."

"Well, I'll quit now."

"Can I have your cigarettes?" I knew her supply was endless; taking them would be like trying to cut off the flow of cocaine with a single arrest. Still, it would be a step in the right direction.

"Take 'em Dr. Martin," she said, confidently. I opened her drawer and took out two unopened packs of cigarettes.

"Can I have the others?" I asked.

"I don't have any more. That's all I have," she said.

I knew this woman. She was not about to quit smoking so easily.

"Now you've got to swear you'll quit smoking."

"I'll swear," she said, with no emotion.

"Then swear."

"I swear." Still no emotion. I reached over and picked up her bible.

"Swear on this," I commanded.

"Why do I have to swear on the bible?" Now her voice was rising. "I *said* I wouldn't smoke. Don't you believe me?"

I knew it. She had no intention of quitting. Unless I could get her to swear on the bible, she would never take her promise seriously. "Mrs. Wiggins you've got to swear on the bible. Otherwise God won't believe you're sincere."

She hesitated and her body began to shake. She looked at me, then the bible, then at me again.

"Dr. Martin," she said indignantly, her voice trembling a little, "that's the word of the Lord! You want me to swear on the Bible?"

"Swear!" I was transforming my demeanor into that of a medical evangelist. "SWEAR!"

"I can't do that!"

"Then you don't intend to quit. You lied to me."

"But I will quit, Dr. Martin. I promise!"

"Then SWEAR ON THE BIBLE!"

Slowly, hesitatingly, she placed her right hand on the bible. I could sense the adrenalin flow. I was about to make my first convert.

"Repeat after me. I, Amanda Wiggins..."

She hesitated and looked at the nurse. Not wanting to break the spell with another voice, the nurse merely nodded her head, affirming my command. Then Mrs. Wiggins looked back at me. My eyes were fixed on hers. There was no way out. She repeated my preamble.

"I, Amanda Wiggins..."

"Do swear before God in Heaven..."

"Do swear before God in Heaven..."

"That I will never touch or smoke cigarettes again."

"Oh, Dr. Martin!"

I repeated the command with raised voice. "THAT I WILL NEVER TOUCH OR SMOKE CIGARETTES AGAIN. SWEAR, MRS. WIGGINS!"

"That I will never touch or smoke cigarettes again," she echoed.

"SO HELP ME GOD!" I bellowed.

"So help me God," she responded. With the last word her whole body shook and she began crying. I checked her pulse and listened to her lungs. No acute problem. She was not having an asthma attack, just a religious experience. Had I reached her? I left Ms. Wiggins sobbing quietly on the bed. The nurse watching the scene promised to check her every half hour.

Feeling quite smug about my effort, I went to see other patients. I remember thinking: to get a patient to quit smoking you must learn to communicate on their level, to search out that part of their psyche that listens to the doctor. Why aren't all physicians this creative with their advice?

A half hour later the nurse called me to return to the ward lounge. "You won't believe this," she said. The tone in her voice punctured my balloon. 'Oh yes I will,' I thought. There in the lounge sat Ms. Wiggins, smoking a cigarette. Relaxed and calm, she looked up at me with not the least hint of anxiety.

"What happened?" I asked, feigning a hurt incredulity. "You PROMISED me you would quit. You promised GOD! You swore on the Bible!"

"I just had to have a cigarette," she said, flashing an innocent smile.

That was the first and last time I tried religion to break a patient's habit.

Comment

In 1964, when the first surgeon general's report on Smoking and Health was published, 40% of adult Americans smoked regularly. Two decades into the twenty-first century the figure is 20%, or about 50 million people. Of the millions who have quit smoking in the past generation, an estimated 90% did so "cold turkey," without the aid of any therapy or drugs or behavior modification. Nicotine in cigarettes can certainly be addicting, However, as

Mr. Tembo demonstrated, once the firm decision is made to quit, it is not all that difficult.

But some people just can't quit, like Mrs. Wiggins, and the patient in the next story.

– END –

11. "Just give me a cigarette!"

Harold Switek has two major diseases, emphysema and paranoid schizophrenia. His lung disease comes from smoking two packs a day for 35 years. Cigarettes did not cause his psychosis, of course. Though "tobaccoism" is a form of addiction and has long been recognized as such by the medical profession, mental illness is not a known complication.

Smoking is distressingly common among hospitalized psychiatric patients. Smoking helps to allay their anxiety, and any attempt to withhold tobacco tends to make for a bad situation. It is almost impossible to get psychotic patients, such as schizophrenics, to quit smoking, and psychiatrists are reluctant to badger them about the harmful effects of tobacco. As a result, although in-hospital psychiatric patients are forbidden to keep matches, smoking is not generally discouraged by the psychiatry staff. To allow smoking but not matches, many psychiatry wards install a permanent cigarette lighter at the nurse's station.

I knew Mr. Switek's case would be difficult the moment I heard from Dr. Janis, his psychiatrist.

"Larry? Hi. This is Nancy Janis. How are you? Good. I wonder if you could do me a favor."

"Sure Nancy, what is it?"

"I have a fifty-year-old man in Weathergill [Psychiatric Pavilion] who's been there two weeks. He's developed a breathing problem and I can't keep him there any longer. They have no medical ward and I'm afraid he needs to be transferred for medical care. Would you be able to take him on MICU?"

"Sure. How bad is he that you want him in the ICU?"

"He has chronic emphysema and we have him on oral meds but he's getting worse. We can't give IV therapy at Weathergill."

"What medication is he taking? Anything that might suppress his breathing?"

"He's had schizophrenia for decades. Poor Harold. He's been in and out of hospitals. I've only had him as a patient the past year. The only thing I can control him with is Thorazine. He's up to 800 milligrams a day but I think that's a safe dose. He might be able to go without it for a while, but he'll eventually need it."

"Oh," I said. "Well, we'll see what he's like. That much Thorazine probably can suppress breathing in someone with severe lung disease. I may have to stop it for a short time."

"What's happening is his emphysema is getting worse. I think he needs IV therapy."

"No problem. When will he arrive?"

"I'll call an ambulance now. He should be there within an hour. I'll make sure they send a copy of his medical records with him."

"What's the situation with relatives? Is he married?"

"No. He lives with his 80-year-old mother. She's all he has. I'll call and let her know."

"OK. We'll call you back if we have questions about his psychiatric management."

"Good. I'll stop by tomorrow and see him anyway."

* * *

Mr. Switek arrived on schedule. Since everything was prearranged, he came right up to MICU, bypassing the emergency room. My first impression was that he didn't look all that bad. My second impression was that he didn't look all that crazy. I was wrong on both counts.

The MICU nurses put him in bed, took his vital signs, and began setting up an intravenous line. I went in with the intern, Dr. Solomon, to begin our examination. Wearing only shorts and a hospital gown open in the front, he appeared short and stocky, with large thighs and arms. His barrel-shaped chest was covered with hair and his abdomen protruded with about twenty-five excess pounds. The transfer record listed him at 185 pounds, 5 feet 7 inches.

His face was big and round, with a crew cut on top, a feature I've always found incongruous in a middle-aged-man. Mr. Switek did not appear particularly anxious or short of breath, but one can be fooled by patients at rest, especially those with chronic lung disease. I have seen patients comfortable in bed who could not walk across the room without gasping for air.

On closer observation his breathing problem was more apparent. Dusky skin and lips signified oxygen deficiency, all the more remarkable because he was receiving oxygen through a nasal cannula. Rapid respiratory rate (34 breaths a minute) and contracting neck muscles signified his dyspnea. His blood pressure was normal, heart rate increased, and temperature up slightly to 100 degrees.

Probably because of his psychiatric history I was also cognizant of some subtle features. His eyes were open wider than normal and he gazed through rather than at you. He did not make eye contact for more than a fraction of a second. Also, his speech was rapid, much faster than the typical patient with severe lung disease.

"Hello, I'm Dr. Martin and this is Dr. Solomon, my resident. How are you?"

"I want to call my mother. Is she here? What's your name? What are you going to do? Is my mother here? Where are my shoes? Why can't I have my shoes?"

"She's been called, Mr. Switek. She knows you're here. And you won't need your shoes while you're in the ICU."

"She wants me home. I want to go home. Where are my shoes? Hey, can I have a cigarette? Where are my cigarettes?" With this last question he began turning his head from side to side and up to the ceiling, as if we were hiding his cigarettes close by, somewhere in the ICU cubicle.

"You can't go home now, Mr. Switek. You were sent here because of your breathing."

"Hey Doc, there's nothing wrong with my breathing. I just want a cigarette. Can I have a cigarette? Where are my cigarettes? I'll just take one."

"That's impossible, Mr. Switek. You're in the intensive care unit! There's oxygen all around you."

"I'll go outside. Can I have a cigarette?"

"Can I listen to your lungs?"

"OK."

Dr. Solomon and I went right to his lungs and heart, bypassing areas customarily examined first. No telling when he might decide not to cooperate. Facing each other behind Mr. Switek's hairy back, Dr. Solomon and I each placed a stethoscope up and down his chest, listening to him breathe. Our eyes met as our ears heard the same thing: diffuse and severe wheezing, sometimes described as "tight breathing" because it signifies air squeezing through constricted passages.

"Better check his blood gases," I said, and Dr. Solomon left to get a syringe for the arterial blood sample. I came around the side of the bed to face Mr. Switek.

"Now can I have a cigarette?" he asked, as soon as he saw me.

"You can't smoke!" I gesticulated, flapping my hands up and down for effect. "You'll blow up if you smoke!" (Not true, but I thought this would get to him.)

"Naaah," he said, without missing a beat. "I won't blow up. You're just saying that. Please get me my cigarettes. Where are they?"

"First let's see what our tests show," I said.

"OK. But I can have a cigarette first?"

MICU could handle any type of lung problem. Could we handle a psychotic patient with a lung problem?

Thirty minutes later we had results of arterial blood gas analysis, chest x-ray, and electrocardiogram. Mr. Switek's oxygen level was barely adequate, only 85 percent despite receiving extra oxygen. The cardiogram showed a heart strain from the low oxygen, and his cardiac rhythm showed skipped beats and other ominous irregularities. Fortunately, his chest x-ray was clear: no pneumonia.

Our diagnosis was acute bronchial infection on top of emphysema, with impending respiratory failure. He was almost at the point of needing intubation and artificial ventilation. Perhaps with an increase in inhaled oxygen, plus antibiotics, steroids and other medication, he could get by without intubation. I went in to tell him the news, realizing he probably wouldn't hear a thing I had to say.

"We have the results of the tests, Mr. Switek. Your lungs are really bad. We're starting treatment with some powerful drugs. If they work, you'll recover from this breathing attack. If not, we might have to sedate you and put a tube in your throat. Under no circumstances can you smoke. Do you understand?"

"Okay. When can I get my cigarettes?"

He was incapable of understanding. It was like talking to a child.

"Look, I'll make a deal with you. Let us treat you for a few days. When you get better you can have a cigarette." Never before had I offered such a deal.

"Okay," he said.

We discontinued Thorazine since the drug was probably depressing his respiratory drive, and continued supplemental oxygen through a nasal cannula. At this point improving his breathing had a higher priority than treating his psychosis.

Over the next 24 hours his blood oxygen level came up a little but his heart beat still danced around the monitor and his wheezing was as tight as before. We vacillated about whether to intubate him and begin artificial ventilation. There are no numbers to go by for such an important decision, only careful bedside observation coupled with the results from arterial blood gases.

During his first 24 hours in MICU Mr. Switek's breathing became so labored that he actually ceased asking for cigarettes. In the middle of the second day his agitation increased, a probable result of not receiving Thorazine. At Dr. Janis's suggestion we restarted the drug at a much lower dose than she had used before, only 100 milligrams twice a day.

On the evening of the second day Mr. Switek deteriorated rapidly. His breathing became more labored, nostrils flared with each breath, and he looked like a fish out of water. Coupled with cardiac irregularities and poor oxygenation, all signs pointed to the need for artificial ventilation. We called anesthesiology.

The anesthesiologist came and injected him with a quick-acting paralyzing agent; without complete paralysis Mr. Switek would have been too difficult to intubate. His neck was too fat and he was too agitated. Once intubated, the ventilator took over his breathing. We then placed an arterial catheter in his arm so frequent blood samples could be obtained for oxygen and carbon dioxide measurements.

Over the next few hours the ventilator corrected his oxygen and carbon dioxide levels. As paralysis wore off, we began sedative medication so he would sleep; he had not had much sleep since arriving to MICU. We held Thorazine while he was under sedation.

With sleep, adequate oxygenation and antibiotics Mr. Switek's condition improved. After two days of artificial ventilation his lungs sounded clear. We stopped the sedation and tested his lung function with the ventilator temporarily disconnected. It was much better. We pulled the tube from his throat.

For the next eight hours Mr. Switek was docile: no complaints, no agitation. Then, towards the evening he asked his nurse for a cigarette. She explained that he couldn't smoke.

"Just give me a cigarette," he insisted.

"Harold, you know you can't smoke. You just came off the ventilator," she reasoned.

He did not argue the point. Instead, he waited for her to leave the room. Then he got out of bed to go search for tobacco. This was not so easy in his condition. Mr. Switek had been in bed for four days, two of them unconscious, narcotized. Anyone in his state should get out of bed slowly and always with assistance.

Incredibly, standing up for the first time in several days didn't make him faint or even cause a wobbly gait. However, he still had an arterial catheter in one arm, connected by delicate tubing to a monitor, and a venous catheter in the other arm, through which he received antibiotics. As he moved away from the bed, each catheter disconnected from its extension tubing. The venous catheter dripped dark red blood. The arterial catheter, being in a high-pressure vessel, spurted blood of a brighter hue.

"Harold, where are you going?" his nurse called out. Harold didn't answer.

"You'll bleed to death," she exclaimed. This was not an idle threat, as arterial blood continued to spurt from the catheter in his arm.

"Naaah. I'll be OK. I need a cigarette." He headed toward MICU's double doors and the EXIT sign.

The nurse quickly realized he was not about to get back in bed. "Let me pull those tubes out of you," she said bravely. He let her. That done, he felt free to roam. Although blood still oozed from the puncture sites, at least he would not exsanguinate.

"I want a cigarette," he said to the night clerk at the nurses' station. She got up and walked away.

Two nurses implored him to get back to bed.

"OK," he said. "Just give me a cigarette, OK?"

"We can't, Harold," they pleaded. "Please get back into bed."

He moved on, a sight to behold, walking around the MICU nurses' station wearing only a hospital night shirt and no underwear, with blood from each arm dripping to the floor. Our schizophrenic patient was unconcerned with his appearance or health or the scene he was causing. He was possessed with a single idea: CIGARETTE! The nurses kept their distance. Finally, one of them called Security. Then me.

Mr. Switek again headed for the swinging doors that separate MICU from the waiting area. No one tried to stop him. He left MICU and walked down the hallway toward the elevators, where he was met by a security team of two large men.

"Where are you going, sir?"

"I'm looking for a cigarette machine." (There is none in the hospital).

"You have to get back to your room, Mr. Switek."

He asked the security guard for a cigarette. They proceeded to escort him back to MICU. As he did not offer any resistance, he may have thought they were taking him to a cigarette machine.

I arrived in MICU just as he was being escorted back by the officers. At the entrance to his room it dawned on him that he wasn't being led to a cigarette machine, and he turned around rapidly to go the other way.

At this point the scene became physical. He had to be restrained to prevent injury to himself. He would have walked in front of a moving car to get a cigarette. The two guards with the help of a male nurse grabbed his arms and pulled him toward the bed. Harold began thrashing around. Leather restraints were yelled for. He was literally lifted up and thrown onto the bed. One arm, then the other arm, then both legs were tied securely to the bed frame.

Within minutes Mr. Switek was in full leather restraints, thrashing around the bed, screaming and crying. It was impossible to keep a sheet on the bed or an intravenous line in his arm. Sedation was out of the question because of his lung condition. And the last thing I wanted to do was intubate him again.

He looked at me and yelled, "You can't do this to me! You promised me a cigarette." He remembered!

"Mr. Switek, we have to do this," I apologized. "You're going to hurt yourself if we don't keep you here."

He began to sob, the sobbing of a child who has been denied promised candy. I left the room and called Dr. Janis. I needed help with this man-child, this schizophrenic, tobacco-addicted, emphysema-riddled bull of a patient. I had to keep him from killing himself.

Dr. Janis recommended trying Haldol, a drug less sedating than Thorazine that can be given by intramuscular injection. I agreed. Controlling his psychosis now took priority over his breathing, which was much improved anyway.

Mr. Switek stayed in leather restraints another thirty-six hours, until the Haldol took effect. Fortunately, his breathing remained stable and he was able to take his other medications orally. On the sixth hospital day the leather restraints came off. Miraculously, he had calmed down and was no longer a threat to himself or others.

"Call my mother," he requested.

His mother, old and infirm, had not been able to visit him in MICU. I wanted to speak with her also, so I brought a phone into his room and dialed the number. I handed over the receiver as soon as it began ringing.

"Ma? This is Harold. I'm still in the hospital. They're trying to kill me, ma. Yeah. They had me all tied up...Yeah, they tried to kill me...Bring my cigarettes, Okay, Ma? I'm coming home now...I don't know, here's the doctor."

I took the receiver from Harold and talked to his mother, a very pleasant lady who, I imagined, had been through some hellish times with her son. She was quite reasonable on the phone. I explained the situation and why her son had to stay in the hospital a little longer and why he could not smoke. She understood and thanked me, adding that she was ready for Harold "whenever you and Dr. Janis say he's ready to come home." We said goodbye and I hung up the phone.

"Okay, Harold. Your mother says she can't come to see you now but knows you're coming home soon."

He started to cry again. I tried to console him, to reason with him, but it was no use. Mr. Switek was ill in ways I didn't understand, and I felt powerless to help. Since he was not in imminent physical danger, I thought it best to just leave him alone.

* * *

The next few days went more smoothly than I expected. We gradually weaned down the Haldol dose and switched him back to Thorazine. An arterial blood gas test showed adequate oxygen and carbon dioxide levels. We allowed him to walk outside his room as long as he stayed within the confines of MICU.

By this time a mentally normal patient would have been transferred to a regular ward, but Mr. Switek's psychosis required that he either remain in MICU or go to a psychiatric ward. On the eighth day of hospitalization he returned to Weathergill. During the entire 170 hours in MICU he did not have a single cigarette.

Follow-up

This episode took place in the late 1980s. I kept in touch with Mr. Switek's medical progress through his psychiatrist for about ten years, then lost track of him. During that period he remained on Thorazine and continued to smoke heavily. He did not need further hospitalization for his lung problem.

– END –

12. Pickwickian

I knew Gloria Fallows for about two years before she was admitted to Intensive Care. I first saw her as an outpatient in 1992 when she was 63. Even then she was enormous: 275 pounds, five feet two inches, and had trouble breathing. Her chief complaint was "shortness of my breath."

"Oh, Dr. Martin!" she exclaimed back then. "I can't walk from here to there without struggling." She pointed to a wall of my office about ten feet away.

"How long, Mrs. Fallows? How long's it been this bad?"

"Only the past few months. But it seems to get worse each day."

Weight was her problem. Imagine carrying a hundred-pound sack of potatoes packed around your abdomen and rib cage. Just like movement itself, your breathing would be *restricted*. Gloria breathed this way all the time. Each of her breaths was limited, too shallow to do a proper job of gas exchange.

We normally take in about half a quart of air with each breath. Gloria could only manage one-fourth of a quart. She needed more air than her chest cage, overburdened with largess, could oblige; as a result, her blood carbon dioxide level was too high and oxygen level too low. Gloria was comfortable at rest but exhausted on walking any distance or climbing stairs. "I get wiped out, Dr. Martin," she would explain.

Breathing problems also interrupted her sleep. She awoke each morning exhausted from incomplete slumber. To compensate, she frequently napped during the day and at the worst times. She'd been in two car accidents after falling asleep at the wheel. No one was seriously hurt, including Gloria, but at age 62 she had to quit driving.

After that first visit, I diagnosed Gloria's problem as typical of Pickwickian syndrome. Like all syndromes, Pickwickian is not a specific disease as much as a collection of abnormal findings. To most physicians the appellation "Pickwickian" connotes a fat, sleepy patient who has some difficulty breathing. A more precise definition is any patient with obesity, excessive daytime sleepiness and elevated blood carbon dioxide pressure (PCO_2). A high PCO_2 in the blood signifies inadequate breathing or, in medical parlance, "hypoventilation."

Many medical conditions are called by the name of the doctor who first described the malady, like Graves' Disease for one type of over-active thyroid (see Chapter 17). Less commonly, the name comes from that of the original patient, an example being Lou Gehrig's Disease (see Chapter 22).

Pickwickian Syndrome is unique, for it is not named after any doctor or patient Pickwick. Instead, the name has a literary pedigree. The term is traced to a common-named character in Charles Dickens' first novel, *Pickwick Papers* (published 1837). At the end of Chapter 53 Dickens introduces a scene involving the fat boy Joe (see artist's rendering):

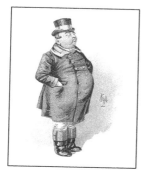

A most violent and startling knocking was heard at the door; it was not an ordinary double knock, but a constant and uninterrupted succession of the loudest single raps, as if the knocker were endowed with the perpetual motion, or the person outside had forgotten to leave off. . .

The object that presented itself to the eyes of the astonished clerk, was a boy - a wonderfully fat boy - habited as a serving lad, standing upright on the mat, with his eyes closed as if in sleep. He had never seen such a fat boy, in or out of a travelling caravan; and this, coupled with the calmness and repose of his appearance, so very different from what was reasonably to have been expected in the inflicter of such knock, smote him with wonder.

"What's the matter?" inquired the clerk.

The extraordinary boy replied not a word; but he nodded once, and seemed, to the clerk's imagination, to snore feebly.

"Where do you come from?" inquired the clerk.

The boy made no sign. He breathed heavily, but in all other respects was motionless.

The clerk repeated the question thrice, and receiving no answer, prepared to shut the door, when the boy suddenly opened his eyes, winked several times, sneezed once, and raised his hand as if to repeat the knocking. Finding the door open, he stared about him with astonishment, and at length fixed his eyes on Mr. Lowten's face.

"What the devil do you knock in that way for?" inquired the clerk, angrily.

"Which way?" said the boy, in a slow and sleepy voice.

"Why, like forty hackney-coachmen," replied the clerk.

"Because master said, I wasn't to leave off knocking till they opened the door, for fear I should go to sleep," said the boy.

Dickens' 19th century portrayal lay medically dormant for over a century, until 1956 when Dr. C.S. Burwell and colleagues published a medical case report, "Extreme Obesity Associated With Alveolar Hypoventilation: a Pickwickian Syndrome." After quoting Dickens' description of the corpulent Joe, the authors went on to describe their patient, a 51-year-old business executive who stood 5 feet 5 inches and weighed over 260 pounds:

[He] entered the hospital because of obesity, fatigue and somnolence. . .The patient was accustomed to eating well but did not gain weight progressively until about one year before admission . . . As the patient gained weight his symptoms appeared and became worse . . . he had often fallen asleep while carrying on his daily routine . . . on several occasions he suffered brief episodes of syncope [fainting]. Persistent edema of the ankles developed . . . Finally, an experience which indicated the severity of his disability led him to seek hospital care. The patient was accustomed to playing poker once a week and on this crucial occasion he was dealt a hand of three aces and two kings. According to Hoyle this hand is called a "full house." *Because he had dropped off to sleep he failed to take advantage of this opportunity.* [Italics original]. A few days later he entered . . . hospital.

. . .Therapy consisted chiefly of enforced weight reduction by means of an 800-calory diet. On this regimen the patient's weight fell from 121.4 to 103.6 kg [267 to 228 pounds] in a period of three weeks. As he lost weight his somnolence, twitching, periodic respiration, dyspnea and edema gradually subsided and his physical condition became essentially normal.

Since that first medical paper thousands of patients have been diagnosed with sleep disorders. The spectrum of problems ranges from occasional insomnia to sleep walking to the far more serious (and potentially life-threatening) Pickwickian syndrome. Today many hospitals run "sleep labs," secluded rooms replete with bed and exotic monitoring equipment for charting physiology during sleep.

Gloria Fallows needed such an evaluation. More importantly, she needed to lose weight. Even if her sleep pattern tested normal, which I knew it wouldn't, her weight was a serious health problem.

Gloria's wedding picture at age twenty-three showed a woman of 140 lbs., solid and attractive. By age fifty, she tipped the scales at 200 lbs. but had no (known) medical problems. At sixty, she weighed 240 lbs. and was under treatment for high blood pressure and diabetes. She added another thirty-five pounds over the next three years. Fortunately, Gloria did not smoke; if she had, the combination of cigarettes and morbid obesity would likely have been fatal well before I ever saw her. As it was, she could barely manage.

Why did she eat all that food?

"I don't eat that much." she said. "Honest I don't, Dr. Martin."

Doctors used to discount this oft-heard claim of the morbidly obese, but to a certain extent it may be true. Body metabolism plummets in late middle age, and a reduced caloric intake may not bring about any weight loss, at least not without the addition of exercise. But daily, aerobic-type exercise for people like Gloria Fallows is seldom feasible. The only solution for most massively obese people is such a drastic decrease in calories that medical supervision becomes necessary.

Gloria had been on diets before, but they always failed. "No will power," she confessed. But she had never been in a medically-supervised weight loss program.

"Gloria," I said, "you need two things. First, you need to lose weight in a special program so doctors can follow your metabolism. And we need to study your breathing to see why your oxygen is so low. The only way to do both is to put you in the hospital."

"Hospital? It's that bad?"

"Yes," I insisted.

"Will my insurance cover it?"

I checked. Her insurance plan did not recognize hospitalization for obesity alone, so I admitted her for "respiratory failure, chronic." Unfortunately for Gloria this was a legitimate diagnosis, confirmed by the elevated carbon dioxide in her blood.

We did a battery of tests to check organ function of her heart, lungs, liver, kidneys, pancreas, and adrenal glands. Surprisingly, all tests were normal or near-normal except her lung function. She had reduced lung volumes, confirming our clinical impression of restricted breathing. As a result of not being able to take deeper breaths, her blood oxygen pressure was only 55 mm Hg (millimeters of mercury; normal is above 80) and carbon dioxide pressure 53 mm Hg (normal is between 36 and 44, with an average of 40). Some physicians jokingly refer to patients like Gloria as belonging to the "50-50 club," signifying the abnormal blood oxygen and carbon dioxide levels. Membership is definitely not desirable.

By the evening of day three our routine tests were completed. We sent her to another wing of the hospital for a sleep study, technically known as polysomnography, the recording of many (poly) records (graphy) during sleep (somno). The study is conducted in a windowless room with the subject asleep on a queen-sized bed, reinforced to sustain the heaviest patients. A technician hooked Gloria's head, nose, ear, chest, and extremities to multiple wires emanating from sundry monitoring devices.

I went to observe the beginning of the sleep study. Lying in bed, wired up, surrounded by all kinds of electronic boxes, Gloria looked like a character in a sci-fi thriller.

Twenty minutes later Gloria was asleep, so I left her to the technician and his monitoring devices. She slept from 10 p.m. to 6:30 a.m., when she was wheeled back to her regular ward bed. I saw her on morning rounds a few hours later.

"Well, Mrs. Fallows, did you sleep well last night?"

"Off and on, Dr. Martin. Off and on. They sure had me wired up."

"How do you feel now?"

"Okay. A little tired, I guess."

I went to the sleep lab to check the results. Gloria's polysomnogram showed three things. She snored a lot. Her throat tended to close and block her upper airway during sleep (a condition called sleep apnea). And, her blood oxygen level fell, at one point to a level incompatible with any longevity. During sleep Gloria Fallows was at risk for *sudden death*.

I prescribed a night-time breathing machine, called "Bi-PAP" for Bi-level Positive Airway Pressure. A Bi-PAP machine is essentially a watered-down version of the full-scale life-support ventilator, the kind used routinely in intensive care units. About the size of a toaster, the Bi-PAP machine sits on a table or night stand, and is connected to the patient via a long hose. At the end of the hose sits a small, nose-shaped mask, made out of soft rubber. With the aid of head straps, the mask can fit tightly over the patient's nose, so air will not escape as it is pushed through the nostrils (older mask versions covered both mouth and nose, but they proved too uncomfortable for night time use).

During sleep the Bi-PAP machine pushes air through the nose, upper airway and lungs. This "pushed" air enters under increased pressure, and in this manner helps prevent the upper airway from collapsing while the patient sleeps. The air pressure is highest on inspiration, when the machine does all of its work. The patient exhales passively and the air pressure falls, but is still elevated above normal; hence the two levels of air pressure. Better ventilation helps transfer oxygen into the lungs and remove carbon dioxide, ameliorating the Pickwickian's gas exchange problem.

When the Bi-PAP machine works, it works well. But it can be uncomfortable. Gloria tried Bi-PAP only two nights before rejecting it. "It's like sleeping in an air vent," she said.

I could not argue, having never slept with the device. For the record, however, many patients gladly accept the machine's incessant WHOOSH-whoosh, WHOOSH-whoosh, in exchange for a night without sleep apnea. Spouses often have a harder time.

I prescribed a more comfortable nasal cannula for use during sleep; through it, extra oxygen enters the nostrils and lungs, but at no increase in air pressure. Though not as effective as Bi-PAP, nasal oxygen at least kept her oxygen level from hitting rock bottom during sleep.

In the middle of week two Gloria started a liquid-protein supplement diet. All solid food was taken away and she drank only the liquid meal, several times a day. The supplement allows the body to burn mainly carbohydrate and fat during what amounts to semi-starvation. For patients who stick to the supplement there is often remarkable, and safe, weight loss.

After three weeks in hospital Gloria went home weighing 255 pounds. A twenty-pound weight loss was not bad in such a short period, but the first twenty are the easiest. Now all she had to do was continue the diet, plus use her nasal oxygen at night.

At first, all was success. A month after discharge she weighed 240 pounds. In another two months she weighed 230 pounds, a satisfying drop of forty-five pounds in only three months. She looked and felt better, and her oxygen level was up.

Unexpectedly, she quit attending the clinic. Since that was the only place to get the protein supplement, she quit dieting as well. About a month after her first missed appointment, I received a card from the weight-loss clinic: "Your patient, Gloria Fallows, has dropped out of the Liquid Protein Diet Program. Please let us know if we can be of any further help in her weight control."

I called her. "Mrs. Fallows, what happened? Why did you quit going to the weight clinic?"

"Oh, Dr. Martin. I couldn't get a ride anymore. And it was just too far by bus."

People who lose weight in the best of programs frequently gain it back. Reasons for sliding are varied, but Gloria's was a common one—some obstacle to keeping the clinic appointments. In her case, she could have found other transportation but didn't make the effort.

On the phone, she admitted to gaining weight and having more trouble breathing. I saw her the next day, in my office at the hospital. She weighed 262 pounds and had much leg edema (swelling from excess fluid). A chest x-ray confirmed early congestive heart failure. I admitted her to the hospital and began diuretics to mobilize the fluid. She did not need the intensive care unit on this admission.

Our specialist in morbid obesity saw her in consultation. He didn't mince words, writing in the chart: "Given the severity of her problem and recent failure on the liquid protein diet, I suggest consideration for gastric stapling. Please contact Surgery."

First you try dieting without supervision. That seldom works. Then you try supervised dieting. That is sometimes successful. When dieting fails, you have a range of procedures to choose from, all disappointing in their long-term results. Gastric stapling, literally stapling the stomach into a smaller pouch for receiving food, was at one time a popular operation for the massively obese. (The "stapled" stomach was supposed to make the patient feel satiated with less food. Success with the operation was limited, however, and is seldom done anymore.)

A surgeon visited Gloria to explain the operation and the risks. "Let me think about it," she said. She thought about the procedure for two days and then decided against it. "I'll lose weight with the diet," she said.

"Gloria," I remarked on learning of her decision, "you failed the diet. You gave up."

"Oh, Dr. Martin! I won't quit next time. I promise."

"It's up to you, Gloria."

"Let me try again."

She was accepted back into the diet program. We also made special arrangements for transportation if she couldn't find a ride to the clinic. Most patients are given only two chances in the program; this was Gloria's second.

She left the hospital in a week, weighing 253 pounds.

* * *

Gloria quit the diet three months later, this time with the excuse that "it just wasn't for me." Compliance is everything in weight reduction and there was nothing more the diet clinic could do.

She continued using the nasal oxygen and diuretic medication, and her weight did not go down. It didn't go up either, but age was against her. What the 40- or 50-year-old-body can tolerate, the 64- or 65-year-old can find unbearable.

I followed Gloria, along with her internist, but we could not correct her underlying medical problems. Her oxygen and carbon dioxide levels remained grossly out of balance. She was a ticking time bomb, and I told her so on more than one occasion. It was a question of when, not if.

The bomb went off in late March 1994, just after she turned 65. I was called from the emergency department. "Dr. Martin, this is Dr. Thompson. I understand you know Gloria Fallows? Her internist asked that I contact you."

"Yes, yes. What happened?"

"Mrs. Fallows came in about an hour ago, almost apneic. We intubated her and will be sending her up to MICU [Medical Intensive Care Unit]."

"I was afraid this would happen. What caused her to fail?"

"We don't know. Chest x-ray's clear, and her cardiogram shows no acute changes. She apparently collapsed at home and EMS [Emergency Medical Service] was called. When she got here, her PCO_2 was ninety-six and PO_2 only thirty-five."

"Wow!" I replied, surprised at the severity of those numbers. "Sounds like she was on her way out."

"Yes," said Dr. Thompson. "We had real trouble intubating her. Finally had to put the tube through her nose. Her blood gases are improving on the ventilator and she's stable enough to be moved. Do you have a bed available now?"

"Sure. Send her right up."

I *thought* I knew Gloria, but the person rolled into our intensive care unit was much larger than what I remembered. She must have gained at least another fifty pounds. Three nurses and two doctors lifted her from the transport stretcher to hospital bed. *Heavy.*

Her MICU bed rested on a scale so that additional weight could be accurately recorded. She weighed 318 lbs. and looked it. Her belly was enormous. How could anyone breathe with all that fat pressing on the lungs?

About thirty minutes later, after things were squared away with our patient, I went to speak with Mr. Fallows in the family waiting area. A thin, balding man in his mid-60s, he had just recently retired from a job with the post office. I knew from previous visits that their marriage was a good one and that Mr. Fallows was devoted to her care. Unfortunately, there was little he could do without her cooperation.

"She's stable now, Mr. Fallows," I said. "But she was in a lot of trouble when she arrived. What happened to her? She's gained a ton of weight since I last saw her."

"I don't know, Doctor Martin. She just lays around at home and doesn't do much. For the last few days she's been kind of mopey. Today I couldn't even get her out of bed."

"Why didn't you call us before?"

"She didn't want to come to the hospital. She told me not to call the ambulance. Said she was fine, just wanted to be left alone."

I affirmed that she was critically ill and could die any time.

"Well, I have faith. Just do what you can for her, Dr. Martin."

Our initial tests did not reveal any acute infection or other explanation for her deterioration. She seemed to have worsened just from increase in both age and weight. That left only weight to correct. Until we took off a couple dozen pounds, or at least redistributed the fat so it didn't squeeze her lungs, she would likely need the ventilator.

The next morning on rounds we found her awake, lying in bed with her head raised slightly on one pillow. She looked pachydermish with the endotracheal tube coming out of her right nostril, a giant, thick neck, and a mountain of fat south of that. Her legs were huge, rounded limbs of hardened tissue, the result of years of waxing and waning edema. The skin around her ankles was bluish-red and scaly.

I arranged the sheets to expose her abdominal protuberance. We've had heavier patients before (one of 550 lbs.), but Gloria's short stature and Jabba-the-Hut appearance made her look more grotesque than the others. Clinical knowledge and professionalism aside, very large patients always elicit a bit of voyeurism. So it was on teaching rounds with the interns and residents. Everyone stared at Gloria's belly.

Placing my hands on her huge abdomen, I pronounced: "*This* is the problem." Mrs. Fallows nodded in agreement. "I'm not going to minimize the situation, Mrs. Fallows. Your weight is killing you. It's got to come off." She nodded again.

"We'll do what we can to get that tube out of your nose. But when we do, you have to lose some weight. No, a *lot* of weight. Or you'll be right back here." I pointed to her bed and she nodded.

I reviewed the ventilator settings and blood gases with the house staff, examined Gloria's lungs and heart, noted her fluid intake and urine output. She was stable but not ready to come off the ventilator. I led the house staff out of her room, to resume discussion near the nursing station.

"What would you do now?" I asked Sherry, one of the senior residents. A petite young woman, she was perhaps the brightest of the group.

"I don't know. Can we keep her on the ventilator while she loses weight? I guess that's one way to stop her from eating."

"Is there any alternative?" I asked the group. "Can we get her off the ventilator the way she is now?"

They were stumped.

"What's her major problem?" I asked.

"Her weight."

"Right. Any other problem?"

"Well, hypertension."

"Right, that's a problem too, but it's not what I'm thinking of. Is there any other reason she could be in respiratory failure besides the weight?"

"She doesn't smoke and has no asthma. Her chest X-ray is clear. What are you getting at, Dr. Martin?"

"Suppose you studied blood gases [measurements of PO_2 and PCO_2] and breathing capacity in twenty non-smokers, all under five feet three inches and weighing over 300 pounds. What do you think you would find?"

"I don't know," said Sherry. "Did you do that study?"

"No, but others have. Breathing abnormalities were found in most of them, but not enough to seriously impair gas exchange. In other words, they did not have frank respiratory failure like Mrs. Fallows, even in those over age 60. The point is, weight by itself is not the only problem. There has to be some other factor or factors to explain *her* respiratory problem. I've been following Mrs. Fallows for two years. Even when she weighed two-fifty, she had hypoxemia [low oxygen level] and CO_2 retention.

"Most likely, patients like Mrs. Fallows have an abnormal brainstem respiratory center. For some reason, her brain won't let her do the extra work of breathing all that extra weight requires. Many obese people *are* able to do the extra work and maintain decent oxygen and carbon dioxide levels. She can't do the extra work necessary for deeper breaths, so her levels remain life-threatening. It's just a theory, but it does help explain why most very obese patients don't have her problem.

"Would respiratory stimulants help?" asked Sherry.

"You mean some kind of pill to stimulate her breathing?"

"Yes, something like that."

"A few have been tried, particularly progesterone. They generally don't work, and if they do it's only over the long term. It's not going to help in the short term. We've got to get her off the ventilator very soon. Any other ideas?"

"What about a fatectomy?" someone else asked. (Literally, cutting off the excess weight.) The question generated snippets of laughter.

"What about wiring her jaw shut?" queried another, eliciting more laughter.

"You laugh, but those are possibilities. Still, you're not really answering my question. How can we safely get her off the ventilator in the next few days?

She's not going to lose enough weight to make a big difference in a few days. How are we going to do it?"

"Diuretics," someone said.

"Diuretics will help mobilize excess water, but probably won't make much of a dent in her belly. Anyway, she's already on Lasix [a potent diuretic]. Any other ideas?"

No answer.

"Well, there's one way," I said. "A therapy too little used in intensive care. What is it?"

They were stumped by my guess-what-I'm-thinking question.

"I'll give you a hint. It's not a drug and not a medical device."

"What else is there?" asked Sherry.

"I'll give you another hint. It's an elemental force of nature. One of the four primary forces."

Ohhhhhhh," swooned one of the heretofore silent residents, a quiet chap who had been listening intently.

"Yes?" I asked.

"Isaac Newton."

"That's right! Very good. We're going to use *gravity*. It's free and every room is equipped. If we don't get that tube out of her throat soon, she's bound to have a major complication. Infection or airway damage. A tracheostomy on Mrs. Fallows would be very difficult. She has no neck. A surgeon looking to place a hole in her trachea could get lost." The house staff glanced back at Gloria, visible through the glass door, and nodded in agreement.

"We've got to get her off the ventilator," I said. "The easiest way to take advantage of gravity is with . . . an anti-gravity bed."

"What's that?"

"A bed that will allow her to sit up without sliding. Look at her. She's in the anti-breathing position, all squinched up in bed. With the typical hospital bed like this one, you can't keep her abdomen from attacking her chest. How can anyone breathe with all that weight squeezing the lungs? If we can just unload her lungs a bit, I think we can get her off the ventilator."

"Marsha," I said to our head nurse, "can we get her one of those Big Boy beds? You know, the kind we used for that five-hundred pound patient?"

"Sure, Dr. Martin. I'll see what I can do."

* * *

Unlike a conventional hospital bed, the Big Boy is constructed in four bendable sections. Each section can be adjusted to place the patient in practically any desired position. The Big Boy made it possible to care for

Gloria in a semi-sitting position, night and day, effectively shifting her massive abdomen *downward*, away from her chest. By using gravity to lower the abdominal mass, her lungs had more room to expand with each breath. She remained in this posture, with slight variation, for the next two days while we gradually turned down the ventilator settings.

On her third day in MICU we disconnected the ventilator. At that point she breathed on her own, but still through the endotracheal tube. Her arterial blood gases remained about the same as baseline values: PO_2 64 mm Hg, PCO2 59 mm Hg. I decided to take a chance and remove the endotracheal tube. We could always put it back in.

After extubation, Gloria's PO_2 remained low, PCO_2 high, but not deranged enough to require re-intubation. Still, she wasn't ready to leave intensive care. She remained in that precarious state I call "ventilator limbo": almost-but-not-quite needing artificial ventilation, almost-but-not-quite ready to leave MICU for a regular ward bed.

When not sleeping, Gloria just lay in bed. She made few demands on the nurses and generally seemed unconcerned about her situation. There was no hint of desire to get better and leave MICU. Had she given up? Or was her moodiness just a result of deranged blood gases? We found no evidence for neurologic damage. She was oriented and conversant but simply unmotivated, listless really. Overall, a bad sign.

* * *

Gloria's fifth day in hospital, April 1, was also the day some of our house staff changed rotations. Gloria got a new intern, Roger Bailey, a 29-year-old with career interest in one of the surgical specialties. Roger was in his ninth month of internship (the academic year begins in July) and had already spent a month in our ICU the previous October. He knew his way around. What he didn't know, unfortunately, was much about pulmonary physiology.

Interns and residents cannot choose their patients. They have to take whoever is assigned on the rotation. If Dr. Bailey had any choice, it would not be Mrs. Fallows, for he was not sympathetic to her medical problems. As far as he was concerned, if she just took deeper breaths she could get out of the ICU and off his service. He did not like obese, slothful patients.

During morning rounds on April 3rd, he asked, "Dr. Martin, can we transfer her out of MICU today? I don't think we're doing much for her here."

"What are her blood gases this morning?" I asked.

"About the same. PO_2 fifty-six, PCO_2 is seventy-two, on nasal oxygen."

I reviewed all the blood gases measured since extubation. They did not show much variation: low oxygen and high carbon dioxide. We had tried

117

everything to increase her ventilation, including the Big Boy bed, deep breathing exercises, adjustments to diet, and diuretics to mobilize edema fluid.

"I don't know," I said wistfully. "I wish she could just take deeper breaths and lower her CO_2 level."

At my remark Dr. Bailey's eyes opened wide. He must have been looking for the proper opening, and I provided it. "I think I have an explanation for her failure to improve," he said, rather professionally.

"Really? What?"

"Mrs. Fallows just doesn't want to breathe more. It's her personality. She needs motivation." Translation: let's get a psychiatry consult and transfer her out of intensive care.

This may seem, to the lay mind, a not unreasonable suggestion; after all, much illness can be related to depression, poor motivation, low self-esteem. But even assuming psychiatry had something to offer by way of remedy, Dr. Bailey's explanation and understanding of her situation were naive, wrong-headed. I decided to respond with mock incredulity.

"*What*? What did you say? The problem's her personality?"

"Yes," Dr. Bailey replied. "Some patients just don't want to breathe deeply. She's just lazy and wants to be this way. Maybe psychiatry can help her."

How to answer this medical delusion? He was so scientifically confused I was actually amused. Personality and attitude have nothing to do with why patients under breathe or have a low oxygen level. First-year-medical-school physiology teaches that one cannot raise carbon dioxide or lower oxygen levels by any aspect of *will or mind control*, transcendental or other forms of meditation notwithstanding. That is why children who hold their breath to gain attention cannot really stop breathing. The brain's breathing control center won't let a child (or an adult) voluntarily slow down ventilation to a dangerous level. As soon as the control center senses the slightest buildup of CO_2, *you will breathe*. It's that powerful a stimulus.

I knew this, but did Dr. Bailey? I decided to give him the benefit of doubt. Perhaps I misunderstood his explanation. "You mean because she eats a lot that her breathing is affected, and that psychiatry could help motivate her to lose weight. Is that what you mean?"

"Well, that too," said Roger. "But you see this kind of breathing in lazy people. It's just her basic personality."

Wow! I thought. This is getting out of hand. Was he serious or just being playful?

"Roger, do you have a reference for that?"

"Well, I read that somewhere," he said lamely.

"Where?"

"I don't remember. Somewhere."

Time to attack.

"Roger, suppose you measured the PCO_2 of everybody with any kind of psychiatric disorder, excluding people on massive amounts of anti-psychotic medication. What would be the average PCO_2 of all these people? Would it be high, low or normal?"

"Oh, I don't know," he said.

"Anybody?"

"Forty?" asked Sherry, my medical resident.

"Right. Very good, Sherry. Forty point oh oh. In other words, normal. And suppose you measured PCO_2 of people who are, say, just depressed and mopey, but not with a bona fide psychiatric diagnosis? What would you find, on average?"

No one answered, so I did, "Forty point oh oh." There was no comment, so I continued.

"And, what's the average PCO_2 of all the people who are nasty, mean, uncivilized, unwashed, or just plain *lazy*?"

This time I waited for someone else to answer. A short pause, then Sherry spoke up once again: "Forty."

"Right again. In other words, normal. Any other bad traits you want to know about as far as the associated PCO_2?" It was all in good fun. No one seemed offended. I liked to think the house staff were enjoying the repartee.

"Roger," I continued, "you clearly don't understand what can make someone under ventilate. Fat can do it. She's fat. Some kind of structural lesion in the brainstem can do it. That's a theoretical possibility here, but there's no way to prove it. Long-term smoking can do it by causing severe lung damage, like emphysema, but Mrs. Fallows doesn't smoke. Some drugs can slow breathing, particularly sleeping pills and narcotics, but she's not on any of those. Weakness of the chest cage muscles can do it, and she may have that problem to some extent. But personality? Never."

No one said anything. Time for my repetition routine. If you can't help the patient, at least teach the house staff. Make a point they likely won't forget, even if you have to act overbearing while doing so.

"Sherry, can a patient's personality explain an elevated CO_2 level?"

At first Sherry looked startled, but she quickly caught on. "No, Dr. Martin. Personality can't be blamed."

"Roger, can the nature of a patient's personality explain an elevated

PCO_2?"

He took my teasing repetition good-naturedly. "No, Dr. Martin, personality can't be blamed."

"Okay. Anybody have any questions?" No one did.

"Well," I said, "I think we've done everything possible for Mrs. Fallows in MICU. Let's transfer her out."

* * *

I wish I had a happy ending, but the outcome for the morbidly obese patient with respiratory failure is seldom good. Mrs. Fallows stayed in the hospital another two weeks. Her attitude improved along with a return to ambulation. On the day of discharge her weight was down 45 pounds and arterial blood gases, though better than in MICU, were still far from normal.

She was given another chance in the special diet program. She stayed with the diet for a few months, then stopped for the third time. Two months later she collapsed at home. Mr. Fallows called Emergency Medical Service and paramedics reached the house within minutes. They found her apneic and began CPR, which was continued during the ten-minute ambulance ride to the hospital. On arrival in the emergency department she had no pulse, except that provided by external chest compressions. Another half hour of CPR failed to restore her heart beat, and she was pronounced dead. No autopsy was performed.

– END –

13. Coma

There is coma and there is COMA. Jack Wilkerson, a 35-year-old accountant, was out for six months and we never knew why. His case was the stuff of tabloids (**MAN SLEEPS HALF A YEAR -- DOCS BAFFLED**) and also the kind that ends up in medical journals ("Prolonged coma of unknown etiology: report of a case and review of the literature").

It happened this way. One day in July I got a call from the emergency room. "Dr. Martin, we have a thirty-five-year-old man who may have encephalitis. He's confused and febrile to one hundred point two. His brother says it began with a headache last night, and this morning he didn't know where he was."

"Has he been tapped?" I asked.

"Yes, his spinal tap is clear, so we don't think he has meningitis. Anyway, he's going for a CT scan and then to MICU."

Apart from the fact that encephalitis is always a serious medical problem, there was nothing particularly unique or startling about this message. We see encephalitis all the time. Because of the potential for disaster, such as respiratory failure, everyone with this diagnosis is first admitted to the medical intensive care unit.

On arrival to MICU Jack Wilkerson did not look ill at all, just a bit drowsy and confused. Of average height and stocky, he had a day's growth of beard and a sweet, round face that tended to stare off into space, both eyes wide open. He was arousable by shaking his shoulders, and actually answered some questions appropriately, but for others his answers made no sense.

"What's your name?"
"Jack."
"Jack what?"
"Jack."
"Where are you, Jack?"
"My brother."
"Anything hurt you, Jack?"
"Yes."
"What?"
"Yes."
"Do you know where you are?"
"Here."

"Where's that?"
"Yes."

And so it went. All we knew was that Mr. Wilkerson had been healthy two days earlier, and that along with his confusional state, he had a fever but no evidence for meningitis (inflammation of membranes surrounding the brain). Instead, the clinical picture suggested encephalitis or inflammation *within* the brain. His vital signs were stable and otherwise he seemed in good physical health.

Additional medical history provided by his brother was not especially helpful. The patient had never been sick before: tonsils out at age eleven, occasional flu syndrome, but no illnesses of any type for about a year. He was a certified public accountant and lived alone. He was unmarried but had no history of homosexuality. Nor was there any history of drug abuse or alcoholism or travel outside the country. In short, nothing to suggest a diagnosis more specific than "encephalitis of unknown cause."

The CT scan of his brain was negative: no evidence for stroke, hemorrhage, or tumor. We ordered blood cultures and many other blood tests; all eventually came back normal or negative. A "toxic screen" of his blood (a test for about a dozen common poisons and drugs people overdose on) turned up nothing except aspirin, and at a level expected in someone using the drug for headache. Urine and feces were examined for infecting organisms; none were found. Blood was sent to the state lab for viral titers; these results would be inconclusive until repeat testing could be accomplished in three weeks to check for a diagnostic rise in titer.

Six hours after admission to MICU Jack became less responsive. His level of breathing remained adequate but his eyes were now closed, a sign of developing coma. A plastic catheter was inserted into his radial artery so arterial blood could be drawn to monitor oxygen and carbon dioxide. Another tube was inserted through his penis into his bladder, to monitor urine output.

Mr. Wilkerson deteriorated rapidly. Twelve hours after he first presented, his breathing became shallow and his blood carbon dioxide level began to rise. Respiratory failure set in. To provide artificial ventilation doctors inserted a foot-long hollow plastic endotracheal tube into his windpipe, and connected it to the ventilator. Until coma reversed, the patient would have to be breathed by machine.

Another tube was inserted through his nose and into the stomach, for feeding. Twenty-four hours after hospital admission, Jack Wilkerson had five plastic tubes in his body and was completely comatose.

We called in two consultants, Neurology and Infectious Disease. "Stage IV coma) possible encephalitis," opined the former. "Recommend continued support. Check titers for possible viral etiology."

The ID specialist was no more helpful. "Puzzling case, not typical of encephalitis in this area. No indication for antibiotic coverage." (Note to medical readers; this case pre-dated current antibiotic therapy for some types of viral encephalitis).

Mr. Wilkerson's coma continued. More doctors came by, to ponder or wonder or offer their advice. It all amounted to the same thing: wait and watch.

The second week came and went, without improvement. The toll was especially hard on Jack's brother. Tom Wilkerson, 38, owned a cabinet shop, had a wife and two kids, and was as close to his brother as any adult sibling could be. Tom's business suffered as he spent hours at Jack's bedside. "When do you think my brother will wake up? Anything new?" Always the same good questions and always the same answer: "We don't know."

The longer someone is in coma, the worse the prognosis. This is not necessarily because the brain is damaged, but because the rest of the body tends to wither from disuse, particularly the arm and leg muscles. Also, bed sores develop quickly unless the patient is regularly turned from side to side.

The many plastic tubes necessary for medical care can also cause problems. The urinary tract becomes ripe for infection with a catheter in the bladder. The endotracheal tube can damage the vocal cords and trachea. Catheters in the arteries and veins tend to cause inflammation and infection if not meticulously cared for and changed frequently. Also, because of inadequate nutrition, body weight almost always falls in the comatose patient. A feeding tube is no substitute for the healthy appetite.

A completely comatose patient requires a small army of nurses and therapists to prevent complications of lying still for so long. Around the clock, people had to turn Mr. Wilkerson from side to side, massage his muscles, change his catheters, oil his skin, feed his stomach. It would do no good to have him wake up only to be crippled by muscle contractions, or missing a limb from hospital-acquired infection, or suffering a giant decubitus ulcer (these things have happened).

Jack's body was well maintained. As for his brain, it had its own agenda. He did not wake up. There was not even a glimmer of improvement. A brain wave test—electroencephalogram—was carried out once a week, but its pattern never varied: "...slow waves consistent with encephalopathy." No diagnosis, really.

At Tom's suggestion, and with our ready acquiescence, a consultant neurologist was called in from another hospital, someone no more qualified than our own staff neurologist but perhaps able to offer a fresh perspective. His conclusion after two hours with the patient and the chart: "Agree with current management. Continue what you are doing."

Mr. Wilkerson's case became part of the hospital's culture. I was no longer met in the hallway with the perfunctory "How are you doing?" but with "How's Mr. Wilkerson doing?"

"The same," I found myself replying each time. "Still sleeping."

By the middle of the third week, when it became clear Mr. Wilkerson was not going to wake up soon, he went for tracheostomy. This operation places a short breathing tube directly through the neck into the trachea, and is routine for patients who require prolonged artificial ventilation. It frees up the mouth and provides for much better oral hygiene. Also, if the patient is awake, he or she can eat while being breathed by machine.

During the fourth week we took out Jack's nasogastric feeding tube. To provide a better conduit for food surgeons placed a rubber feeding tube directly through his abdominal skin into the stomach, a procedure called percutaneous endoscopic gastrostomy (PEG). With both the endotracheal and feeding tubes removed, Mr. Wilkerson looked much more comfortable. Whether he felt that way was impossible to know.

By the end of a month, all his tubes had been changed at least once, some as many as five times. His weight was down from 180 pounds on admission to 147, and holding steady. Every-other-day blood tests showed no deterioration of any vital organ. In short, Mr. Wilkerson was stable, just not recovering from coma.

Repeat viral titers were sent to the state lab. To our surprise, all tested negative; there was no rise in titer of any virus known to cause encephalitis in our state.

Mr. Wilkerson's case was explored in conference after conference at the hospital. The ID people presented his problem in a seminar on difficult-to-diagnose encephalitis. The neurologists found his length and depth of coma worthy of academic discourse. Lung specialists waxed over the subject of prolonged artificial ventilation. Nurses discussed basic care of the unconscious patient, and the physical therapists highlighted the importance of maintaining muscle tone by passive range of motion. The nutritionists talked about feeding the comatose patient and assured us (as we already knew) that, food-wise, Jack could be kept alive "forever."

Emboldened by his survival, yet dismayed by the lack of progress, we decided it was time to experiment. Perhaps something in our patient's blood was causing coma that we could not detect with all our tests. A method is available for "washing" the blood of unwanted proteins, called "plasmapheresis." Had plasmapheresis ever been used before in prolonged coma? Well, no, at least not in our hospital. But it is used successfully in other afflictions of the nervous system, including Guillain Barré syndrome and myasthenia gravis. True, these are disorders of the *peripheral nervous system*, not the brain, but what did we have to lose? What did Jack Wilkerson have to lose? Because the procedure was somewhat experimental, at least in this case, we asked for and readily received permission from his brother.

Three times a week the plasmapheresis device, a bulky machine the size of a console TV, was wheeled into his room and connected via tubing to his arm veins. Blood from one vein entered the machine to be "pheresed," or washed, and a fresh plasma-like solution was instilled back into another vein. Each washing session lasted about two hours. From experience with other diseases, a beneficial effect from pheresis might not be seen for weeks.

We continued plasmapheresis for a whole month, longer than usual in other diseases. Mr. Wilkerson didn't get worse, and he didn't get better. Essentially nothing happened.

Two months into his hospitalization, at the end of the plasmapheresis trial, I noticed a perceptible shift in attitude among the hospital staff. Many now felt that Mr. Wilkerson would never wake up, that he wasn't going to live. This attitude found its way into the hospital chart, among notes of the several consultants still involved in his care: "Prognosis appears hopeless" and "At this point doubt meaningful recovery" and "Poor outlook. Discussed with brother."

No one actually gave up, of course. He continued to receive excellent care. But the clinical and intellectual excitement of the first two months was no longer present, and other patients and other problems took center stage. Jack Wilkerson's coma became more or less an accepted fact, and his problem was pushed "to the back" of the ICU. We continued daily bedside rounds but his blood was now drawn only once a week, a chest x-ray taken only every ten days or so, and the chart notes became less wordy and appeared less often.

"About the same."

"No change today."

"Vital signs stable."

"Agree with ongoing management."

Only the intern, newly assigned each month, wrote comprehensive notes. Everyone else sort of backed off. This change in intensity of care was entirely appropriate. We had done virtually everything feasible and, apart from supporting his ventilation and monitoring bodily functions, as physicians we seemed to have no therapeutic role. If Mr. Wilkerson was going to wake up, it would be on his brain's own timetable.

Tom Wilkerson never gave up. He was at his brother's side daily, talking to him, reading letters, playing the radio. It is a matter of controversy whether comatose patients benefit from stimulation by familiar sounds. Tom had discussed the issue with several laymen and was convinced of the value of audio stimulation. We were more than happy to go along with this and made sure that Jack "listened" to music via headphones at least six hours a day.

Fall came and went. Discussions were held about sending Mr. Wilkerson to a chronic care facility, but his brother was against it. He felt Jack's only chance was to remain in the hospital, in the ICU.

The new year came. We had no plans to move him or change anything, just to continue administering food, fluids, artificial ventilation, and good nursing care. No one expected anything more.

* * *

One day in mid-January, as suddenly as it had begun, Jack's coma lifted. He opened his eyes and looked at a nurse washing his face. I was not there but heard that she cried out, "Jack, you're awake!"

Because of the tracheostomy tube he could not talk even if he remembered how, but he was evidently coherent. He looked around, as if to ask "Where am I?" Everyone came to see and stare. One nurse remarked, not inappropriately, that it was like seeing a dead man wake up.

Suddenly the chart notes blossomed. "Mr. Wilkerson appears to have spontaneously recovered from prolonged coma," wrote the neurologist. "Will repeat EEG."

"Spontaneous remission of non-infectious encephalitis," wrote the ID specialist.

"Remarkable improvement," wrote the intern in her daily note. "Praise God," said Jack's brother, not usually taken to religious commentary. "What made him come out of it?"

"I don't know. No one knows!" I exclaimed. "Let's hope he doesn't relapse." That is always a possibility with encephalitis.

It took another week to get Mr. Wilkerson off the breathing machine, then several more days to get him to the point of standing at the bedside. Remarkably, amazingly, he continued to improve, haltingly at first, then steadily, with each passing day.

After two weeks of aggressive physical therapy he learned to walk again. The whole hospital turned out to observe. And to enjoy.

One day in early February, Jack was wheeled down to the lobby where his brother was waiting to drive him home. Using a cane for balance and helped by his brother and a hospital aid, but walking under his own power, Jack entered the front seat of the car, and the door closed. He had been hospitalized seven months and three days.

Extensive neurologic testing in April revealed no significant deficits. His EEG was read as normal and residual muscle weakness we attributed to prolonged disuse rather than any nerve damage. He returned to his accounting job and reported no problems with memory or calculating ability. By May Jack Wilkerson was back working a 40-hour week.

Several years after admission for prolonged coma, Jack Wilkerson is healthy and well.

Comment

Jack Wilkerson's recall of seven months in the hospital *begins* with his first trip to physical therapy, about a week after he woke up. The entire hospital stay until that point is a blank. He feels lucky to be alive and, like the rest of us, has no idea what happened or why.

Many people cite his case as an example of why doctors should never give up on a patient in coma, but it is often a comparison of apples to oranges. Mr. Wilkerson's problem was coma of unknown cause in an otherwise healthy body. The outlook is very different for many known causes of coma, such as with the patient in the next story, "Cocaine Wins."

– END –

14. Cocaine Wins

Lester Brown was a large man, at least 6 feet 2 inches and 240 pounds. Even asleep he looked menacingly big, someone you didn't want to wake up before he was ready. The day he was brought to the Emergency Department you could have shook and pinched and tickled Mr. Brown and he wouldn't bother you. He had a ruptured blood vessel at the base of his brain.

It started at home. A few minutes after snorting some cocaine, his posterior communicating cerebral artery began to pulsate, causing him to complain of "the worst headache of my life." Seconds later he fell to the floor, unconscious. En route to the emergency department the artery burst, and he suffered a full-blown *subarachnoid hemorrhage*. The loss of an ounce of blood into the surrounding brain tissue relieved the arterial pressure and the hemorrhage ceased, but by then it was too late. Irritating blood washed over the normally smooth brain surfaces where it didn't belong, and in the process shut down his central nervous system, or at least the part responsible for consciousness. Lester Brown lapsed into a deep coma.

Mr. Brown was 41 years old and had been using cocaine for six or seven years. Like all cocaine-related knockouts, Lester's occurred not from a steady accretion of drug but from a single, exciting snort. Within 30 minutes after inhaling the cocaine, he was in our Emergency Department, comatose and intubated, his breathing fully supported by a ventilator.

A CT scan of his brain confirmed the clinical diagnosis. It showed blood everywhere, both within the ventricles of the brain and covering the outside surfaces. From CT scan he was sent back to the ED, where he awaited a bed in MICU [medical intensive care unit] to open up. The ED staff called for both neurosurgery and neurology consults. I also went down to the ED to evaluate him.

His brother, three years younger but equally large and sinister looking as Lester, gave us the history. 'Bubba' Brown made no attempt to hide his and Lester's illicit drug activity. Indeed, he recounted the details as if we knew all along about their habit and drug trade.

"We just did our thing, man, and this happened. We didn't try to hurt no one. We just dealt with dudes we didn't know too well. Shit, man, this could've happened to me. Motherfuckers!" He was plainly angry in a menacing sort of way but, for the moment, his anger was directed elsewhere. I scanned the ED and thankfully noted the two security guards on duty.

Although Lester's hemorrhage was explainable by a sudden whiff of pure coke—a well-documented cause of stroke—his brother believed in a more sinister cause.

"I told him not to buy off those guys," he said, as if I was supposed to know who "those guys" were. "Lester, he didn't think he had enemies. Man, what are you going to do? I can't believe this happened to Lester. Motherfuckers! MOTHERFUCKERS!"

"What do you think they sold him?" I asked, more out of curiosity about the drug trade than belief that the answer would affect Lester's outcome.

"Never you mind," Bubba said. "I know. And they know I know. Is he gonna make it? I mean, that's what I need to know now, Doc, is he gonna make it?"

"It's too early to tell, but it doesn't look good. The neurosurgeon and a neurologist are on their way to see him now."

* * *

It is axiomatic that all patients are treated without discrimination in both the emergency department and intensive care units. The physical space, the level of nursing care, indeed the entire resources of acute care hospitals are the same for all ED and ICU patients. This *equal level* is not always true elsewhere in the hospital, where there can be distinctions between single vs. private rooms, private duty vs. staff nursing, care by private office-based physicians vs. care by salaried staff physicians, etc. In the ED and ICU, it doesn't matter if you are a pauper or king, drug addict or company president (or both). Care is delivered by the same people to everyone, and is based solely on assessment of the medical problems and the available resources.

Notwithstanding equality of care in these areas, most physicians consider drug addicts and dealers the lowest form of life. We accept that they will lie, cheat, steal and, if necessary, kill to get what they want. But in the ED and ICU, the lowest of the low receives the same top-notch care as anyone else, even if their medical problem is 100 percent drug-related. Doctors and nurses often ponder the irony that the life we save today may rob (or harm) us tomorrow.

So Lester's drug habit and reason for coming to the hospital didn't matter. We would have done whatever necessary to salvage his brain regardless of the cause. Unfortunately, there was just very little to offer. Within an hour of arrival to the hospital both neurosurgery and neurology consultants confirmed Lester's dismal prognosis.

Apart from the fact that the neurosurgeon operates, while the neurologist is mainly a diagnostician of nervous system disorders, a principal distinction between the two specialists is the number of words they leave in a consultation note. The neurosurgeon always writes what is necessary in a page or less. The neurologist seldom makes do with less than two pages, and sometimes writes four or five.

The neurosurgeon who consulted on Lester reviewed the CT scan, did a quick physical exam, and then summarized the situation as follows: "Massive SAH [subarachnoid hemorrhage, a bleeding into the brain]. Little hope for survival. Nothing to offer surgically." This assessment took him only about fifteen minutes in the ED.

The neurologist's summary was a bit longer, and was not completed until after Lester had been transferred to MICU. He wrote: "In the presence of deep coma from SAH the prognosis for survival is very poor. Based on data from [the medical literature], patients like Mr. Brown have a 74% probability of dying from SAH. However, given his specific neurologic findings, particularly the absent oculocephalic response [eye movements when the head is turned] and absent corneal reflexes [blinking when the eyeball is lightly touched], Mr. Brown's chance for survival is only 5%, and even then he would in all likelihood remain in a vegetative state. I simply cannot be optimistic because of the size of his bleed and level of coma. Suggest discussion with his family regarding DNR [do not resuscitate] status. Thank you. Will follow."

Eight vs. over a hundred words to say the same thing. Yet both consultants were helpful. The neurosurgeon told us brain surgery was no use, and that Mr. Brown could be transported directly to MICU, bypassing the operating room. The neurologist told us, authoritatively, what to expect and what to tell the family.

* * *

Once ensconced in MICU, Lester had plenty of visitors. It was not easy to know who was related by blood and who by economic considerations. On his very first hospital day I was told he had "one brother and one sister." The next day, two brothers and two sisters came to visit. He had no wife but at least two "girlfriends." The only relatives I felt certain about were Bubba, his younger brother, and their mother, an attractive, well-dressed woman in her early sixties.

To facilitate communication everyone agreed Bubba would be the official spokesperson, and I dealt only with him. Bubba was seldom alone, however; at least a few friends and relatives usually stood nearby during our conversations.

As so often happens in cases where the principal affliction is self-induced, the patient's extended family did not easily accept the drug connection. Notwithstanding Bubba's comments at the time of admission, I had the distinct impression that everyone else thought something amiss had happened to Lester *in* our emergency room. After all, they reasoned, Lester only came in because of a headache, albeit a severe one. "He wasn't that bad when he left home," they commented. "He was always a strong man. Healthy as an ox."

Bubba did little to dispel this line of thinking, either because he could not make good on his promise of retribution or because he would not admit to dangers from snorting coke. I reassured them repeatedly that the care in the ED had been superb, adding that Lester might *not be here now* had the care been less so.

As expected, Lester showed no signs of improvement. Despite full ventilator support, anti-hypertensive medication, and round-the-clock nursing care, he remained deeply comatose and unresponsive.

* * *

By Lester's third day in MICU, his "family" had grown to twelve people, all sitting or standing vigil in the waiting room. Although only two people are allowed in a MICU patient's room at any one time, there is no rule prohibiting an army, if it wished, to camp out in the waiting area.

That afternoon I managed to catch Bubba alone in Lester's room. I told him the outlook was dismal and that neither myself nor the neurologist thought Lester would survive another 24 hours. I quickly added that we would not stop the breathing machine or any other therapy, and that Lester would stay in MICU until he either died or got better.

No way was I going to even hint at a slackening of care or ask for a DNR order, although by this point I felt intensive care was futile. Nonetheless, it was important, to forestall any doubt about our hospital's management, that we continue with full support until the inevitable end.

"Can you come out and explain to our family?" Bubba asked. "They'll want to hear it from you."

I agreed and followed Bubba out to the waiting room. The four or five relatives who were smoking (near a no-smoking sign) put out their cigarettes, and a woman on the phone hung up when she saw us coming. After everyone assembled in a corner of the large waiting area, I began my explanation. I took the direct approach.

"Unfortunately, there's been no improvement in Mr. Brown's condition. The neurology specialist saw him again this morning and repeated another brain wave test. It looks very bad. His brain activity is only one step above what we call totally brain dead. At this point, in all honesty, we don't think he's going to make it."

"You're not giving up, Doc." A command, not a question, from one of

Lester's relatives.

"Absolutely not," I retorted quickly. "I made that clear just now to Mr. Brown's brother, and I promise all of you, we are in no way giving up. But Mr. Brown wanted me to tell you how it looks, and it looks real bad."

"Well, we're going to stay right here until he gets better. Did you find out the cause yet?"

"We still think it's from cocaine," I answered matter-of-factly. "The CT scan of his brain, the cocaine found in his urine, and the physical exam all point to a ruptured blood vessel like we often see in cocaine users." I refrained from using the word *addict.*

"Sometimes this happens just from high blood pressure, but in Mr. Brown we're pretty certain it was the cocaine." I had gone over the likely chain of events several times already. This time I wanted to add, "So all of you should quit using coke," but didn't dare.

One of the young men in the crowd, a brother or friend or business partner, looked straight at me and said, menacingly: "It ain't no cocaine that did this." I didn't respond since his comment wasn't a question.

After answering a few more questions I returned to the ICU. I hoped I would not be on duty when Lester died, but at the same time felt ashamed at my wish. *Somebody* would have to tell his family.

* * *

Lester's blood pressure collapsed the next afternoon. I was there. Futilely, we pumped on his chest and infused pressor drugs, but it didn't matter. His brain was gone. We pronounced him dead at 4:35 p.m.

"Are you going to tell the family?" one of the nurses asked me. She was not asking *if* I was going to tell them, as if that was an option I could pass on. She was asking if *I* was going to take the responsibility or delegate it to someone else, such as a medical resident.

"Sure," I said. As director of the intensive care unit, what else could I say?

I looked at the intern who had assisted with the resuscitation, an innocent fellow named Bob. It would have been unfair to send him out alone, but he had to learn how to give out bad news. That was part of being a physician.

"Bob, why don't you come with me?"

We went out together. Walking toward the waiting area, I mumbled to Bob that the only way to do this sort of thing is to be direct. He nodded in agreement. Lester's family were all very quiet as we walked toward them. I think they suspected Lester had died and were just waiting to hear it from me.

"I'm sorry," I said. "Mr. Brown just passed away."

There were about two seconds of silence, then all hell broke loose. Lester's two girlfriends started wailing and sobbing. His mother began repeating, in a high-pitched sing song, "Oh No! Not my Lester! Not my Lester!" She went on and on, and some of her words were unintelligible, a chant for the dead.

Then the young man who knew "it ain't no cocaine" began pounding the wall with his fist, at which point Bubba tried to restrain him. This action only backfired, as the pounding man became more combative.

Somebody yelled at me, "Say it ain't so!"

I feebly responded. With my head slightly bowed, and in a manner to indicate that it was so, I said simply, "I'm sorry."

Ordinarily I would stick around, answer questions, commiserate with the family, ask for autopsy permission. Not this time. Discreetly, Bob and I retreated back toward MICU. I felt I had done my duty. The family had been forewarned of Mr. Brown's eminent demise, and I had told them as soon as it happened.

On our way back we heard "*WHAM!*" and the sound of broken plaster. The young man had broken away from Bubba and, incredibly, put his fist through the wall. The blow would have floored Muhammad Ali in his prime. Bob and I rushed inside MICU and called Security. I had a dead man inside and a crazy one outside. We could hear the wailing and crying and banging continue. I feared more for innocent bystanders than for myself or the MICU staff. In fact, I felt protected in MICU. They wouldn't dare enter the sanctuary of the critically ill, where Lester now lay in repose.

Fortunately, I was right, but outside MICU it was a different story. I saw none of the action, but learned the details as events unfolded. Less than a minute after my call two security guards appeared. Ordinarily, two guards can take care of almost any hospital disturbance, but in this case they were outnumbered. The young man's anger had infected the group so much that the guards could make no headway. Reasoned discourse was to no avail.

Standard policy is to escort off the hospital grounds anyone causing a disturbance. But how do you escort a dozen wailing, fist-pounding, angry people who have just lost a loved one? Well, you can't. Two more security guards were called up, for a total of four.

A melee erupted. Punches were swung and jaws hit. Fortunately, no one had a gun or the melee would have added to our ICU census. As it turned out, one guard suffered a bloody nose and one relative had his shoulder dislocated. Both were treated in the emergency room.

For a full hour after the noise abated, the MICU staff stayed put. Then our Chief of Security came in to report all was under control and that two officers would be stationed outside the ICU all night. Apparently, one of the group had made some threatening remarks, necessitating the extra protection. There had been one arrest, the relative who struck the guard.

Nothing came of the threats, and MICU soon returned to normal. Two hours after death was pronounced, Lester's body was unceremoniously taken to the morgue.

Comment

Lester Brown was one of many cocaine abusers we treated every year. Famous victims in the 1980s included the college basketball star Len Bias, the professional football player Don Rogers, and the movie star John Belushi. They were the tip of an enormous iceberg of senseless, drug-related deaths.

Cocaine is a "stimulant" drug and not an opioid. Opioids, which are pain-relievers and include prescription drugs Oxycontin (oxycodone) and fentanyl, and illegal heroin, are today the main cause of fatal overdose. In the U.S. in 2016, the CDC reported 63,632 overdose deaths, with 66% from a prescription or illicit opioid.

– END –

15. Crisis and Lysis

[The patient in this story was treated in the early 1980s, for a blood clot to his lungs. The diagnosis was much more difficult to make back then, compared to today, and the story reflects our diagnostic dilemma. All hospitals today have readily available chest CT scans, which are much more reliable in making the diagnosis of blood clots in the lungs.]

"Doctor Martin, I need some help." The call was from Bill Moody, one of our medical residents working in the emergency department.

"Sure, Bill, what's up?"

"There's a patient down here with chest pain, shortness of breath and hypoxemia (low oxygen level). He's in some distress, and I think he might have a pulmonary embolism, or at least that's the only way I can put his story together. He and his wife just came back from Florida. They drove straight through, non-stop, eighteen hours in the car. I want to take him for a lung scan. But I wonder, should I heparinize him first?"

"Don't do anything yet, Bill. I'll be right down."

Well, I thought, here it is again. Pulmonary embolism. One of the most difficult diagnoses to make *and* treat. The great masquerader, undiagnosed in half the patients who have it. And often over-diagnosed in patients who end up having something else. Difficulty in making an accurate diagnosis of "PE" has long plagued physicians, but nowhere is the diagnosis more bothersome than in the emergency department. Make the diagnosis and the patient must be admitted to hospital. Rule out the diagnosis and, frequently, the patient can go home (maybe the chest pain was just indigestion). *Miss* the diagnosis and the patient can die.

The mere suspicion of "PE" is enough to engender anxiety in the medical staff. "I thought Mr. Jones might have PE" justifies ordering costly tests at any time of day or night. "I couldn't rule out PE in Mrs. Smith" explains why an otherwise rational physician might start a patient on dangerous blood thinners. And "I missed a PE in Mr. Harris" raises the specter of lawyers hunting you down for the inevitable lawsuit. Doctors who suspect PE often feel caught between the proverbial rock and hard place.

What exactly is PE? Embolus is from the Greek *embolos*, meaning "plug." If a blood clot forms in a leg vein and travels to the lungs, it then becomes a pulmonary embolus. Part of the blood circulation within the lungs captures the embolus and becomes, literally, "plugged" from the clot. If more than one blood clot travels to the lungs they are called pulmonary emboli.

Blood clots traveling to the lungs—pulmonary emboli—may arise from veins anywhere, but the legs are by far the most common site of origin. Until the clots break off and lodge in the lungs, they are usually silent; only infrequently do they cause any discomfort in the legs from where they came.

Once the traveling clots reach the lungs they can cause pain, shortness of breath, cough, heart palpitations, sweating, and a host of other symptoms. The basic problem is that, given suspicion of a pulmonary embolus, there was no easy way to make the diagnosis, at least with certainty. Sometimes doctors had to treat the patient based on very inconclusive evidence. Standard therapy was and remains intravenous heparin, a potent blood thinner tricky to use in the best of circumstances. Less frequently employed for PE in the 1980s was streptokinase, a drug more potent, and potentially more dangerous, than heparin.

If treatment was easy, pulmonary embolism wouldn't be such a big headache for doctors. For example, patients with viral infections often receive antibiotics because the treatment is easy, even if it is likely to be ineffective. Unfortunately, there is no simple treatment for PE. Because heparin "thins" the blood by interfering with normal clotting, it puts the patient at constant risk of *bleeding*. Of course, heparin also prevents more clots from forming and going to the lungs, but what's the good of that if the patient has a major hemorrhage?

Still, doctors use heparin because it stops existing clots in their tracks and keeps new ones from forming; the body's own defenses are relied on to break up the existing clots, which can take several days. Heparin is certainly adequate if the patient is not suffering shock or breathing difficulty, and can wait for natural defenses to eat away at the existing clots.

But what if the patient is in real distress because of the clots? Then streptokinase is indicated, since it acts directly to break up blood clots. But, because streptokinase is so potent—it dissolves clots good and bad—the patient may be at greater risk for bleeding than with heparin, for example after a surgical procedure. Also, streptokinase has not been shown to give better long-term survival than heparin. Survival with either drug is about threefold over no treatment, which is why some treatment is mandatory if you make the diagnosis. Think of it this way: streptokinase heals the very sick patient quicker than does heparin, but the long-term result, i.e., survival, is about the same.

In any case, the bleeding risks with either drug mandated reasonable certainty about the diagnosis. The major dilemma in our case was about the diagnosis, not the specific type of treatment. Often the choice is between the lesser of two evils: risk of bleeding from treatment vs. risk of more and potentially fatal clots traveling to the lungs.

Why was diagnosis so difficult? Because the symptoms are what doctors call non-specific, and also because there is no fool-proof diagnostic test. Chest pain and difficult breathing, two hallmarks of PE, are also common in heart attack, pneumonia, pleurisy, esophagitis, the flu, muscle spasms, and many other serious and not-so-serious conditions. Physicians can't treat every chest complaint as a pulmonary embolus, but if the diagnosis is present and missed, that patient's *next* clot could be fatal.

Some situations increase the risk for pulmonary embolism: major surgery; prolonged bed rest or immobilization; pregnancy (particularly third trimester); chronic heart or lung disease; and cancer. Pulmonary embolism is rare in healthy, active people, with one major exception: women taking birth control pills, especially if they smoke.

Compared to pulmonary emboli, the majority of heart and lung disorders, such as pneumonia, heart attack, heart failure, emphysema, and lung cancer, are relatively easy to diagnose. By contrast, PE was both missed *and* over-diagnosed frequently. Trying to diagnose PE sometimes seemed like trying to identify a close friend behind an opaque glass door. If you could open the door you would have no trouble; otherwise, you can only guess who is there.

The definitive diagnostic test back in the 1980s involved passing a catheter through the heart and into the lungs, then squirting dye into the pulmonary blood vessels. That test, being invasive and expensive, was hardly routine. Instead, doctors in most hospitals relied on the lung scan, a nuclear medicine test that images the *effects* of the blood clots but not the clots themselves.

The lung scan is a very sensitive test; almost any lung condition can show up abnormal, including asthma, heart failure, emphysema, pneumonia, and so forth. Still, certain patterns on a lung scan favor the diagnosis of pulmonary emboli. Radiologists who interpret lung scans use terms like "high," "low," and "indeterminate" to describe the probability that a given lung scan represents pulmonary emboli and not something else.

Of course, radiologists can only interpret images as they appear on film. The clinician has to incorporate the scan interpretation into his or her own *index of clinical suspicion. Clinical suspicion* is a catchall term for what a doctor suspects after examining and talking to the patient. Essentially, the doctor caring for the patient asks: do I have a high or low clinical suspicion that my patient has a pulmonary embolus? And, given that index of suspicion, how do I use the results of the lung scan?

When all the rigmarole was dispensed with, including opinions from several lookers-on, it came down to something like the outline shown below (PE = pulmonary embolism). It was seldom this simple, but the chart gives an idea of the diagnostic process we endured. The problem was that "another test" was either the highly invasive catheter study, or some less invasive but usually less conclusive study, such as looking for leg vein clots that might break off and go to the lungs.

Would Dr. Moody's patient be difficult-to-diagnose or straightforward? In this scheme dx = the diagnosis of pulmonary embolism.

Scan reading: probability for PE	Clinical suspicion: for the diagnosis of PE ("dx")	What to do for the patient
High	High	Treat for dx
High	Low	Do another test
Indeterminate	High	Treat, or do another test
Indeterminate	Low	Abandon dx
Low	High	Do another test, or abandon the diagnosis
Low	Low	Abandon dx

***

In the emergency department I met Francis Jarvin, a 50-year-old stock broker just returned from Florida with his wife, Sylvia. I was struck immediately by two things: his breathing and his suntan. Each of his breaths was deep and painful, with the pain mostly felt over his right chest. In effect he "splinted" his breathing, checking each inspiration to minimize pain made worse by chest movement; as a result, his breaths were rapid and shallow. A normal respiratory rate is 10 to 16 effortless breaths each minute; his rate was 40. He wasn't in shock or confused, and his vital signs were stable except for the rapid breathing.

He sported a loud Hawaii-type shirt, pink pants and white loafers, hardly the clothes we see in our Midwest patients (during March, no less). He was clean-shaven, with thinning hair and well-manicured features, and sported a deep, even suntan and slight paunch. He could just as well be lying at the beach as on a hospital bed in our ED. The apprehension in his eyes, the too-rapid movement of his chest cage, and an oxygen mask that obscured his nose and mouth told me he was in the right place.

About ten hours earlier, somewhere in Kentucky, Mr. Jarvin first noted chest pain and shortness of breath. He thought it might be indigestion and didn't want to stop in an unfamiliar city "if that's all it was." About an hour later his wife took over the driving. As soon as they arrived home, she drove him to our ED. Given his level of discomfort, I was amazed he'd been able to finish the car trip.

The oxygen mask and breathing problem made it difficult for him to talk. I needed to be quick and direct with my examination, but also try not to alarm him. I asked Dr. Moody to get me his chest x-ray, blood gas report, cardiogram, and emergency room chart.

"Hi, I'm Dr. Martin. I'll be taking care of you upstairs. I just want to ask you a few questions, listen to your lungs and heart, and then you'll go for a lung scan. I understand you just came back from Florida." I spoke as if I was making conversation with an old acquaintance.

"Yes... that's right."

"I know you're short of breath and in some pain. Don't try to talk too much. Just answer yes or no if you can, or nod your head. You drove home by car?" He nodded yes.

"You drove straight through, all twelve hundred miles, except for stopping a few times?" Another nod.

"What's the longest you sat in the car without stopping? Just give me an approximation."

"About... five... hours... I guess. Maybe more." Mr. Jarvin squirmed with chest discomfort.

"Did you ever have pain in your legs?"

He shook his head.

"I understand you're taking some pills for high blood pressure."

"...Yes, my wife has them."

"Calan and Dyazide, is that right?"

He nodded agreement.

"Have you ever been in the hospital before?"

He held up one finger.

"Once?"

"Yes... for hernia... about ten years ago."

"Okay. I'm not going to ask you anything else right now. Just let me check a few things."

Over the next few minutes I examined his heart, lungs, abdomen, and legs, reviewed his vital signs and initial lab results, and developed a firm impression: severe pulmonary embolism.

Dr. Moody came in just as I was finishing. "They're ready for him in nuclear medicine," he said. "Should we start him on heparin first?"

"No," I said. "He's going to MICU [medical intensive care unit] straight from the lung scan. Please call MICU and tell them we'll be there as soon as the scan is finished. Ask Marsha Ligner, the head nurse, to please order up streptokinase and have two hundred and fifty thousand units ready when we get there."

"You're going to use *streptokinase*?" Dr. Moody had not used this drug before.

"If his scan shows what I think it will, that's what he needs. Heparin isn't going to help him much right now. We need to break up these clots right away."

I accompanied Mr. Jarvin to nuclear medicine, located one floor below the emergency department, in the basement. I was nervous about him. What other diagnosis could this be? I didn't know, but we needed the scan to confirm pulmonary embolism and justify using streptokinase. I just hoped he would finish and get to MICU before some catastrophe occurred.

The technician injected his arm vein with radioactive technetium, the material used for showing up the lungs, then set the scanner over his chest. I watched the images as they appeared on the monitor. In healthy lungs, the radioactive material is distributed evenly throughout the open blood vessels and shows up as a pattern of fine dots with no interruptions. Blood clots in the lungs disturb the distribution of radioactivity and cause blank spaces to appear on the scan. When examined along with the patient's chest x-ray, the particular pattern of blank spaces determines the probability for pulmonary embolism.

Mr. Jarvin's scan showed enormous blank spaces, pie-shaped defects in both lungs evident from any angle the camera scanned. When all the camera angles were completed, I said, "Let's go." I didn't need the radiologist to tell me what I already knew. His likelihood for embolism was "high-high."

In another three minutes we were in MICU. It was 2:30 in the afternoon.

"Marsha, do you have the streptokinase?"

"Ready to go."

"Let's hang it."

* * *

Mr. Jarvin needed both streptokinase and reassurance. As the drug began flowing into his arm vein, I explained the situation.

"You do have blood clots in your lungs," I said. "We've begun a drug that should help break them up. You'll probably continue to feel uncomfortable for a while, but you should feel better as the clots dissolve."

"I hope so," he winced.

And so did I. I thought back to Sabrina Johnson, seventeen years old. So young. And I was younger too; it had been a decade since she showed up in our ED. A high school student, Sabrina presented to the ED with a "chest pains," or at least that was what her thirty-four-year-old mother told the triage nurse. This was only three days after a previous hospital stay for therapeutic abortion.

I remember the girl well: a short, obese teenager, cherubic face. She spoke with a limited vocabulary and, perhaps being so young, did not seem particularly apprehensive about being back in the hospital so soon. She had a history of two pregnancies; the first one, just a year earlier, was brought to term. Her infant boy was being cared for by Sabrina's mother while she attended school.

Her mother related that Sabrina's pains were sharp and fleeting, and that was why she brought her back to us. In fact, the pains probably worried her mother more than Sabrina, who was claiming no pain when we examined her. Sabrina's legs were fat, too fat to properly examine for clots, but such exam is usually not useful anyway. Her oxygen level was normal, which it can be with pulmonary embolism. Her cardiogram and chest x-ray were, in the parlance of medicalspeak, "unremarkable," meaning not abnormal in any significant way.

I saw her in the emergency department right after she arrived, and discussed her case with the staff ED physician. What to do? We thought of pulmonary embolism, considered it a distinct possibility, and so ordered the requisite lung scan. But we didn't heparinize her right away, or even consider the use of streptokinase.

She was not in any distress and actually seemed comfortable in the ED. Although "at risk" for PE—because of obesity and her recent pregnancy—it was just three days after her abortion and we didn't want to risk any bleeding unless certain of our diagnosis. Then, too, Sabrina was only seventeen, had no chronic diseases, and her pains could just as well have been pleurisy, a generally benign viral syndrome. In looking back, I would say our index of clinical suspicion was on the high side of low.

So we ordered the lung scan, and while the technicians wheeled her to the basement, I stood around the ED to chitchat with the staff. If Sabrina's lung scan was negative, we would probably send her home; anything abnormal, and she would be admitted to hospital and probably go on heparin therapy.

Ten minutes later we were paged "stat" to the radiology department; Sabrina was now in distress, even before she had been injected for the lung scan. *Acute respiratory distress*: breathing labored, nostrils flaring, neck muscles contracting, unable to speak. Her pulse raced at 140, and worse, far worse, within a minute, as we stood there, she went into shock. No blood pressure! From that point it was all downhill. Two highly trained ED doctors and myself did CPR for one hour and ten minutes, right in the radiology department. We gave both heparin and streptokinase, plus assorted other drugs, but nothing worked. Sabrina was dead. And we knew the diagnosis, even without the scan. In fact, from the moment we saw her in distress we all knew.

The autopsy confirmed a massive "saddle" embolus straddling both main branches of her pulmonary artery and completely occluding the flow of blood from her heart to her lungs. The pains she experienced before coming to the ED were most likely from smaller pulmonary emboli, sentinels sent out to warn of impending doom. Would she have survived if we had treated her right away, in the ED? Possibly, but we'll never know. I do know that since Sabrina Johnson, I am sensitized to this diagnosis, respectful of what massive pulmonary embolism can do and how quickly it can snuff out a life.

* * *

I had spoken to Mrs. Jarvin only briefly in the ED and during her husband's lung scan test. She deserved some explanation, so I went out to the MICU lounge where she was waiting.

I guessed her to be in her late forties. Like her husband, she was also suntanned and dressed for Florida. She sported a bouffant hairdo anchored by heavy silver earrings, and wore pastel pants and a purple jacket. The clothes were flashy but her eyes suggested stress and fatigue. In dress and bearing she reminded me of sleep-deprived travelers stranded at an airport during a winter storm, all dressed up, incongruously, for warm weather. Events are totally out of their control, both the weather and decisions on when the planes will fly. All they can do is wait and hope and commiserate.

"Mrs. Jarvin," I said, "the scan shows massive blood clots, which explains all your husband's symptoms. We've just started the blood thinning medication, and he seems to be tolerating it well."

"This is serious, isn't it doctor? Can he die from this?"

I thought of Sabrina and almost blurted out "You betcha!" Instead, I replied, "That's always a possibility in this condition, and that's one reason he's in MICU, so we can watch him closely. The next few hours will be crucial, but right now he's stable. Why didn't you stop at a hospital earlier, if he was having chest pains?"

"Why? Why?" she said mockingly. "Because he's bull-headed, that's why! I begged him to let me stop. He kept saying, 'We'll be home in a few hours, it's just indigestion. Keep driving.' So I kept driving. If he doesn't make it, I'll never forgive myself."

"What exactly happened when you got home?"

"He could hardly walk. He certainly couldn't lift the suitcases out of the trunk. I thought he was going to collapse right on the driveway. He was sick, really sick. He could hardly catch his breath. It was all I could do to get him back in the car. I drove straight here. Didn't even go in the house. Too bad the kids are away." The Jarvins had two grown children living out of town.

"Well, you did the right thing, bringing him here as soon as possible, that's for sure."

Mrs. Jarvin stayed in the MICU lounge the rest of the afternoon and visited her husband a few minutes each hour. Their suitcases remained unpacked in the car.

In the emergency department Mr. Jarvin's oxygen saturation was 90 percent, a low value considering that he was inhaling extra oxygen from the face mask. The normal level without inhaling extra oxygen is over 95 percent. In patients like Mr. Jarvin we follow both their respiratory rate and oxygen saturation, the latter with a non-invasive "pulse oximeter," a clothes pin-type apparatus that fits comfortably over the finger. A chronology of Mr. Jarvin's course that afternoon:

2:00 - Respiratory rate 40, oxygen saturation 90%
2:30 - Streptokinase begun
3:00 - RR 35, oxygen saturation 91%
4:00 - RR 31, oxygen saturation 92%
5:00 - RR 26, oxygen saturation 93%
6:00 - RR 24, oxygen saturation 94%

At 6:30 I found our patient comfortable, no longer in pain, actually smiling. His wife was in the room. "I feel much better," he said. "I don't know what you used, Doc, but it sure seems to be working."

I was glad we started streptokinase. Heparin would not have acted nearly so fast. If he didn't have a bleeding complication, the prognosis was excellent.

Comment and Follow-up

Streptokinase was approved by the Food and Drug Administration in 1977 for treatment of pulmonary embolism, and has since been supplanted by newer fibrinolytic agents such as "TPA." These drugs have saved countless heart attack and blood clot victims all over the world.

As a class, fibrinolytic agents are less commonly used than heparin in PE because, in some early studies, the drug seemed to cause more bleeding without improving survival. Yet they break up the clots quicker than heparin and are probably *not* any more dangerous. If used properly, and if the patient is not invaded frequently for blood drawing and other tests, the complications are about the same as with heparin. Certainly, if we need to lyse a patient's blood clots quickly, then a fibrinolytic drug (such as TPA) is the way to go. Heparin is just too slow for that purpose.

We continued Mr. Jarvin's streptokinase infusion another thirty-six hours, then switched him over to intravenous heparin therapy. He stayed on heparin for several days, at which point we began Coumadin, a blood thinner taken by mouth. There was no complication from any of the drugs, and he went home on the eighth hospital day.

Mr. Jarvin took Coumadin for three months, by which time he was out of the danger period. He never again subjected himself to prolonged sitting, the condition that led to venous stasis in his legs and formation of the clots.

Their next trip to Florida was by plane.

– END –

16. Extraordinary Care

Helga Bowman was sixty when her life went into a tailspin. Within one week of March 1982, she learned of cancer in her right breast and emphysema in both lungs.

On March 12, she consulted a surgeon for a breast lump. Suspicious right away, Dr. Spivey explained it could be cancerous and that she might need a mastectomy. He biopsied the lump with a thin needle, removing just a few cells for microscopic examination. The next day, March 13, Dr. Spivey received a verbal pathology report: malignancy. He promptly called Mrs. Bowman, told her the diagnosis, and scheduled a mastectomy for March 16. Because of her long smoking history, he also ordered pulmonary function tests and asked her to see me for pulmonary consultation.

Mrs. Bowman came to my office on March 14. A middle-aged, kindly-appearing woman with a big smile, she displayed all the telltale signs of emphysema: raised shoulders; slightly pursed lips; slow gait; and contraction of neck muscles with each breath. Most emphysema patients are thin and she was no exception, weighing 110 pounds and standing five feet two. She wore a plain cotton dress and little makeup, and kept her brown hair brushed straight back.

"Any complaints?" I asked.

"I feel fine, like always," she said. "Just this lump I noticed last week." She pointed to her right breast.

"How long have you been smoking?"

"I started when I was about twenty. Forty years, I guess."

"How much? Would you say a pack a day?"

"Yes, no more than that. But it never caused me any problems."

As she undressed for the exam, I could see she was limited and less agile than other middle-aged women with normal lungs. Her pattern of speech, an occasional pause to catch her breath, confirmed my visual assessment. She would look quite healthy in a family snapshot but not on videotape.

Her emphysema had developed insidiously. Shortness of breath on exertion and a chronic morning cough became such a routine experience for Mrs. Bowman that she considered the symptoms almost normal. "I thought they just happen when you get older," she explained.

Any lung capacity less than 50 percent of normal indicates marked breathing impairment; her capacity was only 42 percent of normal. This measurement, plus the chest x-ray and my examination, confirmed severe emphysema. Lung disease of this degree doesn't preclude breast surgery, but does make one more cautious. Our concern is the general anesthesia, which can cause problems for patients with respiratory impairment. I insisted that Mrs. Bowman quit smoking right away, and also prescribed inhalation treatments and corticosteroids for the two days before surgery.

She took the bad news and my recommendations surprisingly well. There was no denial, self-pity, or remorse sometimes seen in cancer patients. Just the opposite. The thing I remember most from her days before surgery was how *non-depressed* she seemed. Friendly and outgoing, she was the type of person who found something good in every bad situation.

On my visit to her hospital room the night before surgery, I met Mr. Bowman, a 62-year-old retired fireman. Like his wife, he was outgoing and affable. A short, thin man, he had the parched and wrinkled skin of an outdoorsman. Fishing was his passion. "I've spent most of my life outdoors," he said.

"What do you catch around here?" I asked.

"Walleye. The lake's got tons of walleye this time of year. Just caught several last week."

We bantered a few minutes about the hazards of lake fishing, and then I changed the subject to his wife's operation. I again discussed the risks of surgery and asked if they had any questions.

"No," they replied, with Mrs. Bowman adding, "We have faith in you and Dr. Spivey." Mr. Bowman nodded his agreement and that was that.

"By the way, you did quit smoking, didn't you?"

"Oh, yes," she said. "I'll never go back to cigarettes." The way she had accepted my no-smoking advice was a good sign. Whatever there was to do or take that might help, she would comply.

On March 16, Mrs. Bowman underwent a modified right radical mastectomy. The operation required removing her breast, some surrounding muscle tissue, and lymph nodes in the axillary (armpit) area that drain lymph from the breast. Several of these nodes were involved with cancer, indicating the tumor had spread outside her breast. She would need post-operative radiotherapy *and* chemotherapy to achieve any hope of cure.

She recovered from surgery without any problems and had an uneventful hospital course. Dr. Spivey discharged her a week later. In early April, as an outpatient, she began a regimen of twenty cobalt treatments, one each weekday. The x-ray beams were aimed to the region of her absent right breast and right shoulder area.

Two weeks later, after only ten cobalt sessions, she developed a fever. Pus began to drain from her surgical wound. Radiation therapy was stopped and an antibiotic prescribed, but drainage from the chest wall continued. A few days later we re-admitted her to the hospital.

Skin bacteria had taken hold at the site of surgery and caused a deep, bony abscess in the underlying sternum, or breast bone. Despite heavy doses of intravenous antibiotics over several days, the infection continued to spread, eroding almost completely through her sternum. Unchecked, the infection might spread to her heart.

We called in a thoracic surgeon to debride the infection. The pain of deep debridement necessitated it be done under general anesthesia. Her lungs might not withstand another operation, but there was little choice by this point. The infection had to be surgically removed.

At operation, much of her sternum was like mush. The surgeon drained all the pus and removed several loose bone fragments, then sutured the remaining pieces of bone together with wire. The resulting assemblage of remaining sternal bone and wire did not form a solid breast plate. Although the operation effectively treated the infection, it left her with an unstable chest cage.

Mrs. Bowman was returned to MICU, still connected to the ventilator. Although her chest was covered with bandages, I could see the problem. When she tried to breathe on her own, instead of the chest's normal outward movement with each breath, her chest moved *inward*. An unstable chest cage, added to severely weakened lungs, meant she would never be able to breathe without a machine to assist her. The next day, April 10th, she returned to the operating room for a tracheostomy, necessary for patients who require long-term mechanical ventilation.

Despite this major complication, and the reality that her cancer was far from cured, Mrs. Bowman remained cheerful. Metastatic breast cancer, severe emphysema, three operations, and several weeks in hospital did not daunt her spirit. She continued to have faith in her doctors and display a strong will to live, no matter what the setbacks.

At first I thought her upbeat mood was inappropriate, or at least an indication that she really didn't understand all that had happened. Certainly, I would be depressed in her situation and so expected that she would be, if not clinically depressed, at least sullen and discouraged. Not her. This woman, who had two crippling diseases and a material net worth probably less than the yearly income of most doctors, viewed life only from the positive side. She had a good marriage, healthy children and grandchildren, and everything to live for. Why be depressed?

I did not tell her that getting off the ventilator seemed unlikely, though I did convey this news to Mr. Bowman. Instead, I emphasized the positive. "We're going to start chemotherapy. We can't give you any more radiotherapy but the drugs should help control your tumor."

"Good," she said with her lips. The tracheostomy tube prevented speech but her facial expression said, "Let's get on with it so I can get better and go home."

Over the next month we gave her the latest in cancer chemotherapy. She developed complications, first pneumonia, then urinary tract infection, then a stormy course of high fever and sepsis. At one point we thought she would not survive, but her body rallied and the infections were brought under control. She remained cheerful. The same could not be said for her doctors.

The oncologist and radiotherapist decided that she could receive no more cancer therapy and signed off her case. There was no evidence of tumor recurrence, but her fragile state made it impossible to give additional treatments if the tumor did recur.

At the end of a month in MICU, after her recovery from sepsis, I again tried to wean her off the ventilator. As expected, the effort was unsuccessful. Her lungs and chest wall were all but destroyed. Thus it came to be that, two months after the initial diagnosis of breast cancer, Mrs. Bowman lay in a MICU bed as a pure "pulmonary" case—and a disposition dilemma. Where could we send a sixty-year-old, ventilator-dependent woman?

Ordinarily we would have looked for one of the rare nursing homes that accept ventilator patients, but she would not consider it. Neither she nor her husband wanted her to be in a nursing home.

Mr. Bowman had the solution. "I'll take her home with me."

Before Mrs. Bowman's case, all of Mt. Sinai Medical Center's ventilator-dependent patients either died in the hospital or went to a nursing home. I knew that other hospitals had sent one or two ventilator-dependent cases home, but those patients were wealthy. The Bowmans barely made ends meet on Mr. Bowman's modest pension.

Artificial ventilation at home requires an oxygen supply company able to manage the ventilator and someone to care for the patient 'round the clock. The first requirement is easy, since third-party payers will cover the ventilator care at home (it is cheaper than in a hospital). The second requirement is the usual stumbling block. Continuous nursing care is prohibitively expensive, and insurance companies will not pay for it. Family members can theoretically do the job, but who has family that can dedicate to such extraordinary care? As it turned out, Mrs. Bowman did: Mr. Bowman.

I had my doubts. Mr. Bowman was devoted to his wife, but could he alone do the tasks that, in the hospital, require several shifts of workers? We would not discharge Mrs. Bowman until she was stable, but even then she would require almost constant attention. She needed to be suctioned often, given a bed pan when necessary, and fed three meals a day. The ventilator had to be checked instantly if any alarms went off, and calls had to be made if something went wrong.

Yes, yes, yes, Mr. Bowman insisted. He could do whatever was needed. All we had to do was show him what and how. Having no reasonable alternative, we agreed to send Mrs. Bowman home with a ventilator.

It took about a week for the oxygen supply company to set up a ventilator in their home. To make things easier, we insisted on the same model used in the hospital. The company first surveyed the house and decided the only place for the machine was a tiny first-floor den. It could not go into their larger second floor bedroom because the connecting oxygen tanks were too heavy for any area but the basement. To properly connect the ventilator to the oxygen tanks required that the machine be located on the first floor. (Hospitals use a built-in liquid oxygen system with outlets in every patient room.)

After two weeks of discharge planning, during which Mr. Bowman received instruction from therapists and nurses, Mrs. Bowman was ready to leave the hospital. On the trip from MICU to the emergency room, where the ambulance was waiting to transport her home, a respiratory therapist breathed her lungs manually with an AMBU bag. In the ambulance she received ventilation from a portable, battery-operated ventilator. Besides the two ambulance attendants, a nurse and respiratory therapist also came with her. Mr. Bowman followed the ambulance in his car, and I followed in my car. I also took along our head of Respiratory Therapy. This was a first for him as well.

I had never been to her neighborhood and knew only that it was in a blue-collar district about five miles south of the hospital. We followed Mr. Bowman off an expressway exit that I had passed many times before. Less than 500 feet from the exit the ambulance stopped in front of an aging, two-story wood frame house. Across the street was a gas station and a bar.

She lived on the fringe of a poor working-class section of town, in a house that was modest even by neighborhood standards. On the lot next door, a rusting 1960s Ford rested on cinder blocks, its wheels and one door missing. Adjacent to the gas station was a vacant lot packed with half a dozen partly-stripped cars. In the air was the din of the expressway with its high-decibel trucks roaring by every few minutes, and also a pervasive smell of exhaust fumes. Though not a slum, the neighborhood was far from appealing. I looked around and thought: *this* is where we are sending our first home-ventilator patient?

As for the Bowmans, they were glad to be home. Mr. Bowman made no apologies for the place, either direct or implied. "Come on in," he welcomed with enthusiasm.

The attendants took Mrs. Bowman out of the ambulance on a stretcher and, while the nurse bagged her manually, carried her up two concrete steps and into the house. Mr. Bowman directed everyone to her new bedroom, a linoleum-floored space approximately twelve feet square. Its walls were covered with musty, stained paneling and a single window looked out on the freeway exit; in the distance I could see a large green highway sign pointing the way to "Downtown." In one corner of the room sat her bed, really a cot. Next to the cot stood a Puritan Bennett model MA-1 volume ventilator, its hoses arched in the air, ready for connection. What an incongruous sight!

We moved Mrs. Bowman from the stretcher to the bed and connected her to the ventilator. Mr. Bowman fussed with her a little, fixing her pillow and a blanket, while we checked her tracheostomy tube and then connected the ventilator. I turned the machine on. Whoosh! Whoosh! It worked fine. All the alarms were checked. While the therapists gave Mr. Bowman a final review of the machine's functions, I briefly examined our patient. Vital signs were okay, and she was comfortable in her 'new' quarters. Careful planning had made the transition go quite smoothly.

The plan was to have the oxygen company's respiratory therapists visit the house twice a week, and for them to call me with any medical questions or special problems. Mr. Bowman planned to be home full time. He would call for help as needed. On occasion, their daughter might be able to help out, but responsibility for round-the-clock care clearly rested with Mr. Bowman.

Before leaving the house, I walked around to see the other rooms. All were small, musty, and worn. The dwelling was not dirty; the kitchen, in particular, seemed clean, but I remember feeling depressed about the place and wondering why. Every room, apart from being tiny and cluttered—an ironing board, old TV, fishing equipment, and cardboard boxes filled with magazines occupied half the living room— had that worn-out-linoleum look. No matter how hard you cleaned this house, it would always seem tired and old. Was this a proper abode for a ventilator-dependent patient?

A half hour after we arrived, Mrs. Bowman was safely in her bed and stabilized. After making sure everything checked out, we said goodbye and left. Outside, I looked at our chief therapist and he looked at me. We each had the same thought.

"Not very comfortable quarters," he said.

"No, her room at the hospital was bigger."

"Well, her husband's really devoted. He's learned everything we can teach him about the ventilator."

"It's amazing," I said. "You hear some homeowners complain about their crabgrass, or problems with the swimming pool, or their need for a hot tub. The Bowmans don't have a pot to piss in, and he brings her home on a ventilator!"

The external appearance of the house, the freeway-exit location, the size of the rooms, and the interior decor all made for a depressing situation. But Mr. Bowman was not depressed, nor was his wife, the woman with the cancer and emphysema. *We* were depressed. How long could she live under these circumstances? In this house?

* * *

During her two months in the hospital, almost all of which was spent connected to a ventilator, Mrs. Bowman had suffered innumerable invasions of her artery for a sample of blood. We needed the blood to check oxygen and carbon dioxide levels and thereby adjust ventilator settings. I had never cared for any viable patient on a ventilator without obtaining at least one arterial blood sample a day.

We had also ordered numerous chest x-rays and many other tests, even when she was stable and only waiting to be discharged.

I did not know how often we would do *any* tests now that she was home. I didn't even know when I would get to see her again. The oxygen company took good care of the machine, and their technician called me once a week to report on her progress. "She's doing well," he said. "No problems with the ventilator. Mr. Bowman is managing things better than we expected. We just go in and do the maintenance checks." Given her benign course, I saw no compelling reason to make a house visit anytime soon.

About a month after she left the hospital I got a call from her husband. "Her tracheostomy cuff is leaking. I think it needs to be changed."

The cuff is a small inflatable balloon at the end of the tracheostomy tube [lower left of drawing]. It is normally inflated with air to provide a seal inside the trachea. If the cuff leaks and deflates, the ventilator cannot deliver the proper amount of air to the lungs.

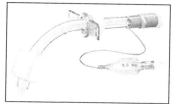

"Is she getting enough air?" I asked.

"Yes, right now she is. But I have to keep inflating the cuff about every hour or the ventilator alarm goes off." Changing her tracheostomy tube was the one thing Mr. Bowman did not feel comfortable doing. It required disconnecting the ventilator for a minute, and that made him anxious.

"Okay, I'll be out this afternoon," I said, and made plans to stop on my way home. Her house was out of the way but I didn't mind. I welcomed the opportunity to help Mr. Bowman, even with a small service. I arrived about 6 p.m. and found her tracheostomy cuff was indeed leaking. I had brought two spares and used one as a replacement.

Mrs. Bowman was all smiles when she saw me. After I changed the tube, she wrote on her pad: "Thank you."

"Are you having any problems?" I asked. "Anything bothering you?

"No," she wrote. "I feel good."

Examination showed that she was about the same as when she left the hospital. Outside, in the yard, where Mr. Bowman preferred to talk, I asked him, "How are you managing?"

"Just fine. I sure am glad you came out. That's real nice of you."

"No problem," I said. "Glad to do it. She seems to be holding up pretty well. Have you been out of the house since we brought her home?"

"No, our daughter Maggie does the shopping, and I just stay here and take care of Helga."

"Can you do this all by yourself?"

"Sure. Maggie helps with the cooking sometimes, but I'm a darn good cook too. We do all right."

Amazing! This man deserves some kind of medal.

Two months went by before I got another call. Same problem. Well, I thought, that seems about right. These trach cuffs last only about eight weeks. I went out to the house and changed her tracheostomy tube.

By my exam, she seemed to be doing well. There were no bedsores that you often see in nursing home patients, and her spirit remained remarkably good. Mr. Bowman was taking good care of his wife. I had thought of bringing a syringe and drawing some blood samples but decided against it. Four months had passed, and nothing untoward had happened. What would I do with the results?

Outside I again asked Mr. Bowman if he'd been able to get away since he brought his wife home.

"I've been to the store a couple of times. Maggie stays with her then, but it's only for a short time."

"Can't you get away more often?" I was concerned about him.

"No. Maggie's got two kids of her own to care for. I'm doing fine," he said.

"Don't worry about me. I don't mind staying home."

I decided to accept what he told me and shut up.

* * *

Over the next two years I made another eight house calls, all to change her tracheostomy tube. I always found her cheerful and appreciative of my visits. She was never out of bed when I came, although I knew she did sit in a chair on those occasions when Mr. Bowman lifted her out. As for her husband, except for an occasional foray to the store, he did not leave the house. He had not gone fishing since we brought Mrs. Bowman home from the hospital.

During those first two years Mrs. Bowman did not have any blood tests or chest x-rays. Word began to spread through the hospital of this indomitable woman at home on the ventilator, in whom not a single blood gas had been drawn in two years. I gave all the credit to the patient and her husband.

One day in August 1984, Mr. Bowman called. "She's got some pain and can't see out of one eye," he said. She had become suddenly blind in her right eye, and his description made me suspect a detached retina.

"Call for an ambulance," I told him. "She needs to be seen by an ophthalmologist."

Two years and two months after leaving Mt. Sinai Hospital, she came back to our MICU. An eye surgeon saw her right away, diagnosed a detached retina, and recommended surgery the next morning. It would have to be done under general anesthesia.

To prepare Mrs. Bowman for eye surgery, I did an arterial blood gas and other routine tests. All the results were normal or unchanged from 1982. The operation was a success and she went home a week later, her vision improved.

* * *

I followed Mrs. Bowman at home for three more years. During this period, I changed her tracheostomy tube about every two to four months. (I always waited for Mr. Bowman's call and then came the same day. I was out of town once and my partner went to the house.) In those three years she had no blood tests or chest x-rays.

One day in June 1987, Mr. Bowman called. "Doc, she's not doing well. Her feet and belly are swollen, and she's falling asleep all the time."

"How long has this been going on?"

"Oh, about a week."

"Does she complain about anything? Any pain or difficulty breathing?"

"No, she just looks bad, Doc, real bad."

"I'll be right out."

I feared the worst but took some diuretic medicine with me in case her problem was uncomplicated heart congestion. Maybe I could treat her at home and keep her more comfortable than she would be in a sterile hospital bed.

Pulling up to the house, I mentally noted the scene: not much different from five years earlier, except that the lot filled with junk cars back then was now vacant, and the Ford on cinder blocks was gone. The expressway hummed as before, and the Bowman's house appeared about five years more decrepit.

Mr. Bowman greeted me as I got out of the car. He repeated his earlier observation. "Thanks for coming, Doc. She looks bad, real bad."

I went to the room and found her very lethargic. I shook her gently and raised my voice: "Mrs. Bowman! Mrs. Bowman!" She smiled and acknowledged my presence, but the old cheeriness was no longer there. Both feet were engorged with edema fluid, but I discerned a different reason for the abdominal swelling. Her liver was rock hard, the first indication after five years that the breast cancer had spread. I went outside to talk to Mr. Bowman.

"I'm suspicious that her cancer has come back," I said.

"I was afraid of that."

"There's little we can do if that's the case. She's had all the therapy possible, and there's nothing else to offer."

"Can she go to the hospital and die there? The grandchildren are always coming over and..." He started to cry.

I fought the same urge. "Sure," I said. "Just wait here. I'll take care of it. Let me make a phone call." I went to the kitchen to use their phone.

After making the arrangements, I returned to Mr. Bowman, who was still outside the house. "The ambulance will be here in a few minutes. I've also phoned the hospital. We'll have a bed for her in the intensive care unit."

"Thanks, Doc." He was still crying.

Follow-up

Our tests confirmed the breast cancer had recurred and spread to her liver. We kept Mrs. Bowman in MICU for two days and then transferred her to a regular ward, where she remained connected to the ventilator and received non-intensive nursing care. We continued intravenous fluids and kept her comfortable with morphine injections. She died in her sleep a week later.

Mr. Bowman accepted the loss. He was grateful for their last years together. After a five-year hiatus, he returned to fishing regularly for walleye. In 1991, when this story was first published, he still lived in the same house, alone, although his daughter and grandchildren visited often.

– END –

17. Thyroid Storm

I'll never forget the patient Roberta Smith, a 35-year-old mother of two who presented to our emergency department with fever, confusion, and a very fast heartbeat. After a brief evaluation in the ED, she was sent to MICU.

As they rolled Mrs. Smith into MICU on a stretcher, I could *see* her problem. Set inside a thin face of smooth and shiny complexion were eyes that bulged like a frog's. A large mass straddled her windpipe, and neck veins on either side pulsated rapidly with the rhythm of her heart. She manifested the classic picture of an extremely overactive thyroid gland, so extreme as to deserve the appellation "thyroid storm."

I examined the ED ledger and x-rays while the nurses put her to bed. The admitting diagnosis was actually pneumonia, with "possible hyperthyroidism" a secondary diagnosis. On chest x-ray, her pneumonia showed up as a hazy shadow in one lung.

There is no test comparable to an x-ray for diagnosing a "hyper"- or over-active thyroid, which is why the ED doctor hedged his diagnosis. Laboratory confirmation is based on blood tests that take much longer to process than any x-ray. Since hyperthyroidism is rarely life-threatening, doctors always wait for blood results if the patient is not acutely ill. In cases in which the diagnosis seems apparent *and* the patient is toxic, treatment is begun immediately.

I asked Mrs. Smith a few questions, but she did not answer. Instead she just stared at me with eyes bursting out of their sockets and moaned: "*Ummmmmmmmm… Ummmmmmmmmmm. Ummmmm… Ummmmmmmmmmm.*"

How had this woman gone untreated for so long?

* * *

The thyroid gland straddles the trachea or windpipe. Although the gland is normally not visible, it can be felt in some people as a slight bulge in the neck area on either side of the windpipe. Mrs. Smith's thyroid gland was at least triple normal size and easy to see. Size alone doesn't indicate over activity; some of the largest thyroid glands, or goiters as they are called, are inactive. Mrs. Smith's gland was both big and overactive.

Thyroid hormone regulates the body's metabolism. When there is too little hormone the patient is said to be "hypothyroid." Hypothyroid patients frequently complain of feeling sluggish and fatigued. They are also intolerant of cold temperatures tolerated by people with a normal thyroid gland.

People with too much thyroid hormone—the hyperthyroids—are often nervous, jittery, and have a fast heartbeat. The most extreme cases of thyroid imbalance, high or low, represent a medical emergency.

Mrs. Smith's clinical exam when she first presented reads like a textbook case of hyperthyroidism:

- Skin warm and moist
- Temperature 102 degrees
- Pounding heart, rate 150 per minute
- Wide, bulging eyes showing twice as much white sclera as normal (medical term: exophthalmos)
- Large thyroid gland
- Muscle weakness in all extremities
- Muscle reflexes 4+ (hyperactive)
- Fine tremor in both hands
- Intolerant of heat (does not keep bed covers on)
- Displays emotional lability; in a span of only 20 minutes from un-responsive and moaning to smiling euphoria to crying to lying quiet.

Another name for her medical diagnosis was Graves' disease, a disorder of altered immunology in which the thyroid's production of hormone is unchecked by normal feedback mechanisms. As is often the case with acutely thyrotoxic patients, she had probably suffered "smoldering hyperthyroidism" from Graves' disease for many months. Pneumonia then pushed her over the brink and into a state of severe thyrotoxicosis, or "thyroid storm."

In the spring of 1991, President George H.W. Bush developed a cardiac arrhythmia from previously undiagnosed Graves' disease. Two years earlier, Mrs. Bush also was diagnosed with Graves' disease. Familial association, i.e., Graves' disease among blood relatives, has been long known but occurrence in spouses is rare. Certainly the disease is not "catching" or communicable. In any event their hyperthyroidism was a much milder form than Mrs. Smith's thyroid storm.

* * *

Robert James Graves was an Irish physician who lived from 1795 to 1853. He is known mainly for his classic paper on hyperthyroidism, published in the *London Medical and Surgical Journal* in 1835; a portion of this paper is quoted below. (From Ralph H. Major, M.D., *Classic Descriptions of Disease*, 3rd Edition, 1945. Courtesy of Charles C. Thomas, Publisher, Springfield, Illinois.)

NEWLY OBSERVED AFFECTION OF THE THYROID GLAND IN FEMALES

I have lately seen three cases of violent and long continued palpitations in females, in each of which the sample peculiarity presented itself, viz. enlargement of the thyroid gland, at all times considerably greater than natural, was subject to remarkable variations in every one of these patients. When the palpitations were violent the gland used notably to swell and become distended, having all the appearance of being increased in size in consequence of an interstitial and sudden effusion of fluid into its substance...

A lady, aged twenty, became affected with some symptoms, which were supposed to be hysterical. This occurred more than two years ago; her health previously had been good. After she had been in this nervous state about three months it was observed that her pulse had become singularly rapid. This rapidity existed without any apparent cause and was constant, the pulse being never under 120, and often much higher. She next complained of weakness on exertion, and began to look pale and thin. Thus she continued for a year, but during this time she manifestly lost ground on the whole, the rapidity of the heart's action having never ceased. It was now observed that the eyes assumed a singular appearance, for the eyeballs were apparently enlarged, so that when she slept or tried to shut her eyes the lids were incapable of closing. When the eyes were open, the white sclerotic could be seen, to a breadth of several lines, all around the cornea...

Since the disease is named after Robert Graves, the grammatically correct spelling should be Graves's disease. However, almost all modern medical texts, as well as unabridged dictionaries, spell it Graves' disease.

Graves' disease is an "autoimmune" condition, which means the patient's own antibodies attack some portion of the thyroid gland, altering the normal regulation of thyroid hormone production. This may be the mechanism, but it does not explain the basic cause. Why do some people generate antibodies to their own thyroid? We just don't know. Stress was once thought to play a role, but that is just a conjecture, never substantiated.

Graves' disease afflicts an estimated one million Americans every year, with women much more commonly afflicted than men. Usually the patient with Graves' hyperthyroidism has a benign course and can be treated as an *outpatient*. What made Mrs. Smith's hyperthyroidism so special was its *rapid and severe* presentation.

* * *

The account by Graves was soon followed by that of Carl A. von Basedow, a German contemporary. Basedow's article appeared in a German medical journal March 28, 1840, part of which is quoted below. (From Ralph H. Major, M.D., *Classic Descriptions of Disease*, 3rd Edition, 1945. Courtesy of Charles C. Thomas, Publisher, Springfield, Illinois.)

> Madame F., brunette, well built, of a decided phlegmatic temperament [married and had four children]. Madame F. felt herself very exhausted, suffered from an obstinate diarrhoea, had night sweats, lost a great deal of weight; at which time the eyeballs began to protrude from the *Orbita*. The patient complained of shortness of breath; she had a very rapid, small pulse; a resounding heartbeat, she could not hold her hand still, spoke with a striking rapidity; and she liked to seat herself (because she always felt burning hot) with naked breasts and arms, in a cold draft. She showed unnatural excitement and carelessness about her condition. She went around a great deal, without being at all disturbed about her striking appearance in company. She satisfied without any afterthoughts her various strong appetites, slept well, however with open eyes.
>
> Sometime in 1837 however, all of these symptoms increased in intensity...in the neck there appeared a strumous swelling of the thyroid gland; the area of pulsation of the heart was now broadened, pointing to enlargement ...the hastiness of speech and the unnatural excitement of the patient still more increased, night sweats, very offensive; urine scanty and read and, considering the continued diarrhoea, the appetite was always too strong. As far as the eyes were concerned, they were pushed out so far that one could see below and above the Cornea...the eyelids were pushed wide from one another; could not be closed with every effort. The patient slept with eyes entirely open.
>
> ...For a long time, the rumor was widespread in our town that this patient was crazy and was soon going to be taken to an asylum, and in fact she had an unfriendly attitude towards the physician; she never had, however, and that I can assure you, any insane ideas; she never showed any abnormal desires and if her astonishing carelessness over her truly sad condition seemed to be the result of her phlegmatic temperament, so the hastiness of her speech, the uncertain holding of her body and her hands, the tendency to go about naked or very lightly dressed, were undoubtedly symptoms of her heart disease.

Graves did not describe any treatment for his three patients. Basedow, for his well-built brunette, first administered leeches, then "spring waters" with "marked improvement." Based on modern understanding of hyperthyroidism, *no* nineteenth century therapy could have been expected to benefit the patient.

For decades after their original accounts, hyperthyroidism was known as *both* Graves' and Basedow's disease. The preeminent clinician of the late 19th and early 20th century in this country was William Osler, one of the founders of Johns Hopkins School of Medicine. In the first edition of his comprehensive textbook of medicine, published in 1892, Osler wrote:

EXOPHTHALMIC GOITRE (GRAVES'S DISEASE; BASEDOW'S DISEASE).

Definition. A disease of unknown origin, characterized by exophthalmos, enlargement of the thyroid, and functional disturbance of the vascular system...The disease is rare in men. Worry, fright, and depressing emotions preceded the development of the disease in a number of cases.

Symptoms. In the acute form the disease may develop with great rapidity. In a patient of J.H. Lloyd's, of Philadelphia, a woman, aged thirty-nine, who had been considered perfectly healthy, but whose friends had noticed that for some time her eyes looked rather prominent, was suddenly seized with intensive vomiting and diarrhoea, rapid action of the heart and great throbbing of the arteries. The eyes were prominent and staring and the thyroid gland was found much enlarged and soft. The gastrointestinal symptoms continued, the pulse became more rapid, the vomiting was incessant, and the patient died on the third day of the illness.

Treatment. Medicinal measures are notoriously uncertain... Treatment of the thyroid gland itself is rarely successful, and the operative measures have not been very satisfactory.

In the United States today, the disease described by Osler is known only as Graves' disease. In Europe "Basedow's disease" is the preferred eponym.

The first effective treatment for any cause of hyperthyroidism was surgical removal of the gland, an operation called thyroidectomy. Although it was not very successful in Osler's time, by the 1920s, with better control of infection and bleeding, thyroidectomy was accepted treatment for large goiters, including those associated with hyperthyroidism.

The first effective drug therapy was inorganic iodine, dating from 1923. In small amounts inorganic iodine stimulates thyroid production, but in large amounts it causes the opposite effect, a lowering of thyroid hormone. Initially, inorganic iodine was used only to prepare patients for thyroidectomy; the operation is less risky if the patient's thyroid gland is first put to rest.

In the 1940s both specific anti-thyroid drugs and radioactive iodine were introduced, making it possible to treat hyperthyroidism *without* surgery. One of the specific anti-thyroid drugs, propylthiouracil or PTU, is still widely used today.

Although PTU and inorganic iodine block overactive thyroid function, they are not definitive treatment. If the patient stops the medication, hyperthyroid symptoms usually recur. To cure hyperthyroidism the gland must be ablated. Ablation can be accomplished either surgically or by radioactive iodine (RAI).

RAI comes as a liquid preparation that is swallowed by the patient. The radioactive iodine enters the blood and is taken up by the thyroid gland, where it destroys active thyroid cells. As a result, the gland shrinks in size. Most patients who take RAI ultimately become *hypo*thyroid within a few years. Fortunately, *hypo*thyroidism is easier to treat than *hyper*thyroidism, so RAI remains an accepted and well-tolerated therapy.

In summary, there are three different methods for treating hyperthyroidism: long-term anti-thyroid medication, such as PTU; RAI, a liquid that is swallowed once; and surgery. Each therapy has good and bad features. Generally, radioactive iodine is avoided in women of child-bearing years. Surgery is preferred if the patient is non-compliant with taking medication. In middle-aged, compliant patients, either RAI or anti-thyroid medication is preferred. (Both President and Mrs. Bush received RAI therapy.)

Ultimately the decision as to which type of therapy to use is based on the patient's particular circumstances and the experience of the treating physician.

* * *

I reviewed Mrs. Smith's case with Dr. Joel Stanley, one of the MICU interns.

"Joel, have you ever seen this before?" I asked, referring to her thyroid disease.

"Graves' disease? Yes, I've seen Graves' disease, but nothing like hers."

"They started penicillin in the ED," I noted. "That's probably okay for her pneumonia. They also drew all the necessary thyroid function tests. We'll get those results in a couple of days, but we have to treat the hyperthyroidism now. What do you want to give her?"

He pulled out his spiral-bound book of intensive care therapy. "Let's see. They recommend several possible treatments."

"By the time you read that book she could be much worse," I replied, in a friendly manner. He was certainly right to research the proper therapy, but she needed treatment right away.

"Joel, while you're reading, let's give her one milligram of intravenous propranolol."

"They mention propranolol," he said, pointing to a paragraph in his book.

"Good. I hope so. It's probably the best thing to use initially in thyroid storm. Propranolol doesn't treat the hyperthyroid gland directly, but it'll slow down her heart. Then we can work on the thyroid gland itself."

Mrs. Smith's heart was in danger of failing from too rapid a rate. Propranolol, a popular cardiac drug also known as Inderal, is excellent for modulating an extremely fast heartbeat.

"What do you want to give next?" I asked him.

"The next step should be an anti-thyroid drug."

"Right. Let's start propylthiouracil, two hundred milligrams every four hours. We'll have to put it down a nasogastric tube. I don't think she can take anything by mouth right now. What else besides PTU?"

"Well," he said, "I suppose we ought to add some inorganic iodine."

"Good idea," I said. "Let's start potassium iodide. Put five drops in some orange juice and put it down her NG tube every six hours."

Iodine is part of thyroid hormone. Giving the drug in its inorganic form helps block thyroid hormone release from the gland. Since inorganic iodine works more quickly than any other anti-thyroid drug, we usually give it to the sickest patients, starting about one hour after the PTU.

After we began Mrs. Smith's treatment, I went out to look for her family. No one was around. Apparently, her husband had left the emergency department as soon as she was transferred to MICU. A call to the phone number listed on the ED sheet went unanswered.

Two hours later, Mr. Smith showed up at the hospital. I explained his wife's condition and told him she was receiving treatment for both pneumonia and hyperthyroidism. Then I asked, "How did she get like this?"

"What do you mean?"

"Well, hyperthyroidism rarely comes on all of a sudden, without any warning. How long has she been so sick?"

"I don't know," he confessed. "She hasn't been feeling well for a while. She's had some diarrhea and headaches for about a week, but we just thought it was the flu. She made an appointment to see a doctor, but that was for next week. Then last night she started coughing and running high fever. This morning she couldn't get out of bed to help our older kid get ready for school. She said she didn't feel well. I got him off to school and then went to check on her. She acted like she didn't know me, and that's when I noticed that funny stare in her eyes. I got scared and just picked her up and brought her here."

"Have you noticed her eyes getting more prominent? Bulging?"

"Well, yes, now that you mention it. But only in the last couple of weeks."

"What did the doctors say when you first brought her in?"

"They talked to me for a few minutes and said her problem was pneumonia and maybe an overactive thyroid gland, just like you said, and that she had to go to intensive care. They said she'd be okay, but she had to be watched very closely. I still had the baby with me, so I left to take her to the sitter's, where she is now. Then I came back."

"Has your wife ever had a thyroid problem before?"

"No, not as far as I know. But she has been kind of high strung for the past year. She saw a doctor about six months ago, and he gave her some Valium, but we never knew it might be from this thyroid gland. At least he never said anything about it."

* * *

By the next morning Mrs. Smith was much improved. Her pulse was down to 110 a minute and she was coherent. A follow-up chest x-ray showed clearing of her pneumonia, so penicillin seemed to be the right antibiotic. In another 24 hours she was able to leave MICU.

Follow-up

Mrs. Smith's pneumonia continued to improve and she stayed in the hospital only three more days. Blood tests begun on the day of admission confirmed a markedly overactive thyroid gland. Potassium iodide was discontinued at the time of discharge. For the next several months, she took only PTU for her thyroid disorder.

Despite PTU, she continued to experience intermittent symptoms from hyperthyroidism. After six months of PTU, her endocrinologist decided to administer radioactive iodine. Fortuitously, the Smiths planned to have no more children. As expected, the RAI obliterated most of her thyroid gland, and she became *hypo*thyroid several months later. Thyroid hormone replacement was started as soon as her gland's output fell below normal. She never suffered symptoms of hypothyroidism.

She continued on synthetic thyroid hormone, one pill a day. Her eyes decreased in size considerably, although they remained somewhat prominent. Most importantly, she was satisfied with her appearance and felt completely well.

– END –

18. As High as a Giraffe's

The top line on Harold Boykin's emergency room ledger was cryptic: "31-yo bm w/cc severe ha and blurry vis p. wk. Hx from wife." [Thirty-one-year-old black male with a chief complaint of headache and blurry vision over the past week. History obtained from patient's wife.]

The first step in ER triage is to obtain a chief complaint and take vital signs: pulse, respiratory rate, blood pressure. Adele, the ER triage nurse, checked Mr. Boykin's pulse at a regular 80 beats per minute, respirations at 18 per minute. Both were normal. To take his blood pressure, she wrapped a cloth cuff around his upper arm and placed her stethoscope bell just below the secured cuff. She placed the other end of the stethoscope in her ears and pumped up the cuff to register 200 mm Hg. [Millimeters of mercury, the units for blood pressure. Hg is the chemical symbol for mercury.]

This procedure is routine for taking blood pressure. At 200 mm Hg, the brachial artery in the arm is occluded, and no blood can get through. With slow deflation of the blood pressure cuff, blood begins to flow through the artery and you can hear this movement with a stethoscope placed over the arm. What you hear is the gentle knocking sound of blood pushing through the partially constricted vessel with each heartbeat. At *that* point, the cuff pressure equals the patient's higher or *systolic* blood pressure, normally between 120 and 140 mm Hg. With further deflation of the cuff, blood flows more freely through the fully-opened artery, and the sounds become inaudible; *that* point represents the patient's lower or *diastolic* blood pressure, normally around 70 to 80 mm Hg.

At 200 mm Hg there should have been silence over Mr. Boykin's arm, but Adele heard the gentle 'knock-knock-knock' of blood rushing through. This meant Mr. Boykin's systolic blood pressure was *higher* than 200. How much higher?

"Let me try again," she said, and she deflated the cuff to restore the circulation. Then she pumped the cuff up to 225 mm Hg. Again she heard: "Knock-knock-knock."

Adele deflated and then re-inflated the cuff for a third try, this time to 250 mm Hg. "Knock-knock-knock." Such an incredibly high pressure! Somewhat in disbelief, Adele looked at Mr. Boykin: "Sir, are you okay?"

Harold Boykin did not answer. Outwardly he appeared healthy: tall, strongly built, good complexion, no indication of any illness, acute or chronic. Yet in response, he simply stared past the triage nurse, awake, eyes open, seemingly unaware of her question. Mrs. Boykin, who had been standing nearby, saw the surprised look in Adele's face.

"Nurse," she asked. "What's wrong? What's wrong with my husband's blood pressure?"

Adele did not answer right away. Instead she reached for the intercom. "Dr. Randall, come to triage, please. Dr. Randall, triage, *please!*"

* * *

The blood pressure of a giraffe is the highest of all animals, reaching about 300 mm Hg in its systolic, or upper phase, and 200 mm Hg in its diastolic, or lower phase.

Normal *human* blood pressure rises with age: around 120/70 for young adults, up to about 140/90 for people over 65. A blood pressure consistently above 140/90 signifies hypertension in most people. How *much* the pressure is above 140/90 is used to classify the hypertension as mild, moderate, or severe and to determine treatment.

The giraffe's blood pressure is higher than ours because the giraffe's heart has to pump blood up a neck seven feet long to reach his brain. The human brain, being only about 12 inches above the heart, is quite nicely served by a much lower blood pressure.

All blood pressure measurements are recorded relative to mercury, a dense element thirteen times as heavy as water. If your blood pressure is "120 over 70," the pressure in your arteries will support an enclosed column of *mercury* 120 mm Hg high in the systolic phase, and 70 mm Hg high in the diastolic phase. These values can also be related to water, which is much closer to blood's density than is mercury.

To summarize blood pressures in the giraffe and human:

GIRAFFE
- Average distance between adult brain and heart = 7 feet.
- Normal blood pressure = 300/200 mm Hg; this pressure will support a column of *water* 3900 millimeters high (12.8 feet) in the systolic phase and 2600 millimeters high (8.5 feet) in the diastolic phase.

HUMAN
- Average distance between adult brain and heart = 12 inches.
- Normal blood pressure = 120/70 mm Hg; this pressure will support a column of *water* 1560 millimeters high (5.1 feet) in the systolic phase and 910 millimeters high (3 feet) in the diastolic phase.

Give the giraffe a human's blood pressure, and the animal will die in a state of shock, unable to pump blood to its brain. Give a man a giraffe's blood pressure, and he will, if death does not come quickly, at least sustain widespread organ damage.

* * *

So-called malignant hypertension—blood pressure high enough to cause damage early in life—has a much higher prevalence in blacks than in other racial groups. The Boykin family has been particularly hard hit. Harold Boykin's father died of hypertension-related heart disease at age fifty-eight. An older brother was under treatment for the same problem. A sister was hospitalized for severe hypertension (eclampsia) during two pregnancies.

Mr. Boykin became aware of hypertension at age twenty-one, his last year of Army service, when a Medic told him his pressure was high and to "take some pills." He finished his Army duty and was honorably discharged. For the next five years, he attended a Veterans' Hospital medical clinic for blood pressure checks and medication. Control of his pressure was erratic, and there were frequent adjustments of medication, yet all the while he felt well. The last drug prescribed affected his libido and was his "last straw": too many medications, intolerable side effects, and all for a disease that didn't make him feel bad. Disillusioned, He quit attending the clinic and stopped all therapy.

Twice after leaving the veterans' clinic, Mr. Boykin showed up in Mt. Sinai's emergency room for flu-related symptoms. On each visit his blood pressure was taken and found elevated, and he was advised to attend our hypertension clinic or return to the VA. Twice he ignored the advice.

Then, at age thirty-one, some six years after his last regular therapy for hypertension, he developed a severe headache. He made no connection between the headache and high blood pressure, especially since he found some relief with aspirin.

A few days later he complained to his wife of blurry vision *and* persistent headache. Still no connection. Mrs. Boykin actually called the hospital's eye clinic for an appointment, thinking her husband might need glasses. The next day his headache became intolerable, and she drove him to Mt. Sinai's emergency room.

* * *

His blood pressure in the ER was finally measured at 280/180 mm Hg, one of the highest recorded in our hospital. Under Dr. Randall's direction, the ER nurses did an electrocardiogram, drew blood, and began treatment with under-the-tongue nifedipine, a drug that induces an immediate lowering of blood pressure.

165

Fifteen minutes after receiving nifedipine, his blood pressure was slightly lower, 260/160 mm Hg. In another fifteen minutes it was 250/150. At that point, he was transferred to MICU.

On arrival to MICU Mr. Boykin appeared in good physical shape, albeit confused. He made no eye contact and did not talk or respond to questions, suggesting swelling of the brain, a potentially fatal condition known medically as *hypertensive encephalopathy*.

We found other stigmata of severe, sustained hypertension: tiny hemorrhages in the back of his eyes (the retina); a large, bounding heart; and protein in his urine. Neurologic exam did not reveal any evidence for stroke or brain hemorrhage, but we ordered a brain CT scan to be sure. Blood drawn in the ER showed diminished kidney function, and his electrocardiogram helped confirm an enlarged, hypertrophied heart muscle (cardiomegaly). The damage sustained by his eyes, heart, kidneys, and brain reflected an enormous arterial pounding: the blood pressure of a giraffe in the body of a man.

We started an infusion of *sodium nitroprusside*, the most potent anti-hypertensive agent available. Nitroprusside directly dilates the arterial blood vessels and almost never fails to lower blood pressure.

Because it is so potent, nitroprusside is a tricky drug to use. If it lowers blood pressure too much, the patient can go into shock from *hypo*tension. If nitroprusside doesn't lower blood pressure enough, the patient will remain at high risk for stroke, heart attack, or kidney failure. The goal of nitroprusside therapy is not a normal blood pressure, but one that is "safely elevated," something on the order of 160/100 mm Hg. The drug's manufacturer cautions:

> [Nitroprusside] should be used be used only when the necessary facilities and equipment for continuous monitoring of blood pressure are available.

"Necessary facilities" means an intensive care unit and round-the-clock nursing care. "Equipment for continuous monitoring" usually requires threading the patient's radial artery with a thin catheter. The catheter is connected via plastic tubing to an electronic monitor so arterial pressure can be continuously recorded and digitally displayed at the patient's bedside.

We began infusing two micrograms of nitroprusside per kilogram body weight each minute, notated in the chart as "2 ugm/kg/min." Within an hour Mr. Boykin's pressure fell to 240/130 mm Hg; within another two hours, 230/122 mm Hg. Still high but safer.

Intravenous nitroprusside is impractical for long periods and is also potentially dangerous. A metabolite of the drug, thiocyanate, is a cyanide-like compound that can starve the body of oxygen. Cases have been reported of cyanide toxicity from prolonged nitroprusside infusion. We planned only a short course.

The next day Mr. Boykin was awake but still not communicating. On a nitroprusside dose of 3.5 ugm/kgm/minute, his blood pressure was down to 200/110 mm Hg, still elevated but not life-threatening. We started him on oral anti-hypertensive drugs and began lowering the nitroprusside dose.

* * *

Most of the 20 million hypertensives in the country never require hospitalization for high blood pressure, let alone intensive care. At Mt. Sinai two to three percent of our MICU patients come in for severe hypertension. They are either 'new' hypertensives, i.e. previously undiagnosed and often with occult kidney disease, or "known" hypertensives, patients who have been non-compliant with prescribed medication.

If a patient is compliant in taking medication and receives good follow-up in the clinic or office, blood pressure can usually be controlled. In fact, some patients improve with just a change in life style: weight loss, no smoking, low salt intake, and exercise.

As to drugs, there are many, many choices, from the tried-and-true to the new-and-exotic. Paradoxically, an explosion in the number of medications in has made treatment both easier and more complicated. Easier, because therapy can now be tailored to the individual patient; more complicated, because the sheer number of drugs makes it difficult for doctors to keep up with their nuances and side effects.

A *single* drug is usually prescribed for mild to moderate elevations of blood pressure. *Two or more drugs* are used for severe cases or when hypertension doesn't respond to a single agent. The actual dose of any drug depends on the patient's tolerance and response. Given the type and number of available drugs, plus the range of dosages, hundreds of outpatient regimens can be formulated.

* * *

By the middle of Mr. Boykin's second day in MICU, we were able to stop nitroprusside infusion and continue therapy with just two oral medications, Catapres and Lasix. His brain CT scan showed no bleeding or stroke, so we expected decent recovery from the encephalopathy.

By day three, his blood pressure was 170/105, and the encephalopathy had cleared. For the first time in four days, Harold Boykin was alert *and* oriented. I had my first discussion with him that afternoon.

"How do you feel?" I asked.

"Much better," he said, without affect. In fact, I was struck by his lack of emotion on this point, certainly none of the glad-to-be-alive attitude we see in some patients. Either he was sullen by nature or perhaps still somewhat depressed by the encephalopathy.

"Mr. Boykin, do you know what happened?"

"I guess my blood pressure was high. That's what the nurses tell me."

"How long have you known about your blood pressure problem?"

"They found it when I was in the Army. That was about ten years ago."

"Do you know how serious it is?" With that question, he looked at me for a few seconds, as if to say, 'What do you think, I'm some kind of jerk?' and I felt a little self-conscious asking these leading questions.

"I guess pretty serious. I wouldn't have all these tubes in me if it wasn't." He still had an arterial line and a venous infusion catheter.

He didn't object to my questions, so I decided to press ahead. "Mr. Boykin, you almost died from your high blood pressure. As it is, your heart is enlarged and your kidneys show some damage. It also affected your brain, which is why you don't remember much about what happened."

His attitude remained rather sullen. He had evidently heard such threats before. Now I was telling him *faits accompli*; these things had happened. His other doctors hadn't been kidding all these years.

"Will they get better?" he asked, with about as little emotion as if one asked "Where is the men's room?"

"We don't know yet. Your pressure's only been under control a short time now. We have to wait and see if any of the damage is reversible. That might take several weeks. You won't stay here in the ICU, of course. You'll have to start coming to the clinic regularly. We'll give you an appointment. By the way, why did you stop taking your medication?"

"I didn't have any to take."

"I mean several years ago, when you were being treated."

"I don't know. That was a long time ago. I remember the medicine made me sick. Sick to my stomach. I actually felt better without it."

"Your wife told me you also smoke."

"Yes, I do."

"How much?"

"About a pack a day. Maybe a little less."

"How long?"

"Since I was a teenager."

I paused for a few seconds. Staring him in the eyes, I said: "I don't know if anyone's ever told you before, but you're a walking time bomb."

"What do you mean?"

"Well, what usually kills hypertensive patients like you is a heart attack or a stroke. You came very close to having a stroke the day you came in, do you know that?"

"Now that you tell me I do."

* * *

I don't enjoy preaching to patients. So many of them are sick because they drink or smoke too much, or use illicit drugs, or don't take their prescribed medications. My Boykin's problems, tobacco addiction and hypertension, are in theory preventable or treatable, like alcoholism and cocaine abuse. Stop drinking, stop smoking, stop abusing drugs. It all sounds so simple *in theory*. The reality is far different.

Intensive care specialists take pride in bringing a diabetic out of coma or rescuing a hypertensive from the brink of death or weaning a patient away from artificial ventilation. The pride may be justified but we should ask on each occasion: would the coma, encephalopathy or respiratory failure have occurred in the first place if there were better outpatient care, more patient education, effective drug rehab programs?

It is one thing to treat an acute, life-threatening illness and another to prevent the problem in the first place. The latter is the real challenge. Compared to providing good outpatient care for patients like Mr. Boykin, i.e., compared to effective *preventive medicine*, intensive care is easy.

Follow-up

On the fourth day in MICU Mr. Boykin's blood pressure was down to 160/95, and we transferred him to the regular ward. He stayed another week in the hospital.

Unfortunately his kidneys were irreversibly impaired, almost to the point of requiring kidney dialysis. A hypertension specialist took over his outpatient management and prescribed a regimen to help preserve remaining kidney function. The regimen included a low-salt diet and three anti-hypertensive drugs: Catapres, Lasix, and Minipress.

Perhaps frightened by events, Mr. Boykin has become very compliant. He regularly attends the hypertension clinic and takes his medication. He knows that blood pressure pills are the only thing keeping him from a suffering a stroke, heart attack, or life-long kidney dialysis.

– END –

19. The Red Baron

Hemoptysis. HE-MOP-TUH-SIS. The word means "coughing up blood," one of the most frightening of medical symptoms. Five quarts of blood speed through our lung capillaries every minute, ceaselessly, until we die. The meshwork of capillaries circle and envelope each of the lungs' 300 million air sacs, so that blood is never far from fresh air. All that separates lung blood from lung air is an extraordinary membrane of microscopic thinness and gargantuan proportion. Stretched out in its entirety the membrane's surface area would cover the surface of a tennis court.

Through this diaphanous barrier gases transfer both ways. Fresh oxygen goes from the air sacs into the capillary blood, to be delivered to the rest of the body; unwanted carbon dioxide goes from the blood into the air sacs, and then exhaled. This vital transfer of gases (oxygen in, carbon dioxide out) is *the* function of our lungs.

Another, separate flow of blood delivers oxygen and nutrients to the lung tissues themselves. Thus, the lungs contain two supplies of blood, one to take up oxygen for the whole body and give off carbon dioxide, the other to deliver oxygen and nutrients to the lung tissues. This is a complicated affair, but it works beautifully. Physicians hardly ever think about the body's dual blood supply (except in medical school!). If either blood supply leaks through the capillaries, the person coughs it out and then there it is: *bright red blood*.

Hemoptysis is scary, but by no means is it always serious or life threatening. There are several grades. "Mild" hemoptysis may occur from just severe coughing; sometimes people "hack" so hard that capillaries rupture and spill small amounts of blood into the large air passages. The blood gets mixed with phlegm and is expectorated (doctors call this "blood streaking"). The problem invariably goes away when the coughing stops.

"Moderate" hemoptysis describes the situation when the patient coughs up a mouthful or so of blood, but not on a continuous basis. The blood may be expectorated once or twice a day. This patient will usually be hospitalized and undergo investigation with x-rays and other tests. Frequently, a bronchoscope is inserted directly into the lungs to investigate the site of bleeding. The goal is to find out not only the cause of hemoptysis but exactly where the blood is coming from (top of the lungs? bottom?).

"Massive" hemoptysis is life-threatening. Blood is coughed up in such quantity, or so frequently, that the patient is at risk of dying from shock or from flooding the lungs with blood and suffocating. Sometimes the patient requires emergency surgery to remove the bleeding lung.

Bronchitis is the most common condition associated with mild hemoptysis. Moderate to severe hemoptysis may be due to a variety of other diseases, including blunt trauma to the chest, pneumonia, tuberculosis (TB), throat and lung cancer, pulmonary embolism, and some unusual "autoimmune" diseases. In the nineteenth century the most common cause of hemoptysis was TB, then known as "consumption" because of the body wasting seen as the disease progressed. Since the 1950s TB has been a treatable condition, and is now a rare cause of hemoptysis.

* * *

When Joseph McShane, 38, came to our emergency department (ED) one Monday in April 1990, his complaint was, "I have hemoptysis and severe pain." Right away this was unusual. Patients don't use medical terms unless they are medical professionals or, as is sometimes the case, their disease is chronic, and they have learned the lingo of their illness. Mr. McShane drove himself to the hospital and was in no distress despite his pain, so the hemoptysis was not considered life threatening.

Except for the most critical cases, who are whisked by ambulance attendants directly into the treatment room, ED patients are asked to state their complaint to a triage nurse. She (or he) is trained to write down the response verbatim, no editing, along with the patient's blood pressure and pulse on an intake form. The nurse is also trained to know who needs to be seen right away and who can wait. Mr. McShane was seen right away.

(Roger Bennett, the ED physician who first evaluated Mr. McShane, later told me of his surprise at seeing "hemoptysis" on the intake form under CHIEF COMPLAINT. His first thought was that Julie Bernstein, the triage nurse that morning, must have shortened the patient's convoluted symptoms into more easily understood medical jargon.)

About 5'10", 150 pounds, Mr. McShane had the lithe build of a long-distance runner. He was dressed in neatly pressed street clothes, no tie or jacket. His physique, coupled with dense straw-colored hair, blue eyes, tan complexion, slightly sunken cheek bones, and a straight aquiline nose bespoke an overall healthy appearance. Looks can be deceiving, of course, and no one who recently coughed up blood can be considered in good health, at least not until the problem is resolved.

"Hello, Mr. McShane, I'm Dr. Bennett. What happened?"

"I woke up this morning and felt OK initially. Anyway, I went to the bathroom and felt some pain right here [pointing to his left lower chest], then something in my throat, like a lump. Then I coughed up a half cupful of blood.

I got scared. I'm from out of town, here visiting my sister, so I don't have a local doctor. Instead I drove right to the hospital. I've had this hemoptysis before, so I knew what was happening and what to do about it." (Yes, that's exactly what he said. At that point Dr. Bennett silently exonerated his triage nurse.)

"Oh? Where? When did this happen to you before?"

Mr. McShane provided a reasonably cogent medical history. He told of two previous admissions to Mercy Hospital in his home town of Atlanta, six months apart, each lasting several days. He had undergone all sorts of tests during each hospitalization. He produced a letter typewritten on Mercy Hospital stationery, dated December 15, 1989; it was signed in longhand.

To Whom It May Concern:

Mr. Joseph McShane was in Mercy Hospital August 1989 with acute pulmonary embolism. His lung scan is abnormal and diagnostic of pulmonary embolism. For acute attacks he receives heparin and coumadin. He can have severe pain with this problem. This letter is being given to him in case he travels out of Atlanta. [Signed, Dr. Howard Lee].

(Pulmonary embolism (PE) occurs when blood clots form in the leg veins, break off and travel to the lungs. PE can cause chest pain and hemoptysis. Heparin and coumadin are blood thinners used to prevent more clots from forming and potentially killing the patient. Heparin is given by vein in the hospital, as soon as pulmonary embolism is diagnosed. Coumadin is an oral (tablet) blood thinner, used for outpatient therapy. PE is also discussed in the story "Lysis and Crisis.")

After reading Mr. McShane's letter, Dr. Bennett asked: "Is Dr. Lee your regular treating physician?"

"Yes. Since the last time I was in the hospital. The first time I had another doctor and she just diagnosed bronchitis. Gave me antibiotics, which probably did no good. I think she missed the diagnosis altogether. Then I got the same symptoms again, and thank goodness for Dr. Lee, he diagnosed the problem. 'No doubt,' he said. You have pulmonary embolism.'" At this pronouncement Mr. McShane winced, either from chest pain or the thought of the wrong diagnosis again being made.

"How long did you take the coumadin for?"

"In the hospital they gave me heparin, and also Demerol for the pain. After a few days the pain went away, and I didn't need Demerol any more. Altogether I took coumadin for about six months, between five and seven point five milligrams a day. This dose kept my prothrombin test [a measure of proper blood thinning] in the therapeutic range."

"So when did you take your last dose of coumadin?"

"About four months ago, in early January."

"And you've had no hemoptysis since then?"

"No, I've really felt fine. Until this morning."

"What kind of work do you do?" Dr. Bennett thought Mr. McShane might be a nurse or hospital worker, given his apparent grasp of medical terminology.

"I'm a computer salesman. I was in the area for business reasons, and when I come up here, I always stay with my sister and her family."

Mr. McShane's physical examination was normal except for two findings. He had a fast heartbeat, or pulse, a common abnormality seen in a hundred different conditions, including ordinary anxiety. A fast pulse is like fever; it generally means something's wrong, but the cause could be just about anything. Mr. McShane's electrocardiogram was negative except for displaying the fast heart rate.

The other abnormality was pain in his left lower rib cage whenever he tried to take a deep breath. We always ask patients to "take a deep breath" when we listen to their lungs. He could not. Midway through a deep breath he would wince, grimace, and stop. Doctors call this sign "splinting" because the chest cage is splinted by pain; the patient cannot fully expand it. The cause is usually pleuritis, which is inflammation of the lining of the lungs (the pleura).

The next test obtained in the ED was a chest x-ray. The x-ray machine is kept in a small room just off the side of the main examining area. About a minute after his x-ray was taken and before he could put his shirt back on, Mr. McShane coughed up a hunk of bright red blood. Having no towels or sink nearby, he coughed the red glob into his shirt. Alarmed, the x-ray technician called for Dr. Bennett to come take a look. Dr. Bennett came, looked, then paged me.

I was in the ED five minutes later and found Mr. McShane holding his side, wincing, in apparent pain. I introduced myself.

"Dr. Bennett told me a little of your history. Are you in a lot of pain?"

"Yes, Dr. Martin, I am . . . Could I have something for the pain?"

I checked the record. He had been in the ED about 35 minutes and had not received anything for pain, which was apparently becoming more severe and frequent. I ordered an injection of Demerol.

Despite the pain and fast pulse, he did not require ICU care, although if he continued coughing up blood, that could change. I learned that he did not smoke or drink alcohol and had no obvious risk factors for pulmonary embolism, such as chronic heart disease, a history of prolonged immobility, or any clotting disorder. He was married and had two children, all back home in Atlanta. He had come to the ED alone, he said, and asked that we not call any family members about his condition. He did not want to worry anyone. Such a request is not unusual and is routinely honored unless the patient is in critical condition.

I formally admitted him to the hospital on my service. Naturally, my first thought was that he had suffered another pulmonary embolism. The sudden onset of coughing up blood and chest pain practically equals pulmonary embolism until proven otherwise. Because the treatment is not easy—long-term blood thinners are tricky to manage—physicians are obligated to prove the diagnosis with some certainty; this is accomplished using one or more tests.

His chest x-ray was normal, which is not an uncommon finding in pulmonary embolism. Clots and inflammation usually cast no shadow on the chest x-ray, unlike pneumonia, which always shows up as a shadow on the x-ray film.

I next ordered some blood work, then sent him for a lung scan. A lung scan is the basic screening test by which doctors diagnose pulmonary embolism. Radioactive material is injected into an arm vein and then imaged by a scanner placed over the patient's chest; emboli in the lung show up as holes or defects in a sea of radioactive dots. (The scan is a little more complicated than suggested by this brief description; see pages 154-155.)

During the hour it took to complete the lung scan, I wondered how we were going to diagnose a new lung clot in a man who already had old clots. The scan would be abnormal, for sure, but it would be difficult to separate new clots from old. Oh, well, I reasoned, it probably didn't matter. Anyone who has a pulmonary embolism once can have it again, and coughing up blood is reason enough to resume treatment. I would have to put him back on his blood thinner, this time for an indefinite period. He would also need a letter to take back home. I had his entire hospital course mapped out, and the letter dictated in my head: "Dear Dr. Lee," it began. "Your patient, Mr. Joseph McShane, was recently hospitalized at Mt. Sinai for recurrent pulmonary emboli..."

But things don't always work out as we expect. An obvious diagnosis sometimes doesn't pan out. A safe assumption is occasionally proved wrong. Whatever the explanation for diagnostic overconfidence, suffice to say that Mr. McShane's lung scan turned out normal, pretty much ruling out pulmonary embolism. At first, I didn't believe the verbal report when the radiologist called, but it was true; I looked at the lung scan myself.

I next arranged for an ultrasound study of his legs. This is a sophisticated test that can actually visualize clots in the leg veins, by sending sound waves through the skin and checking how they bounce back from veins deep within the thighs. An abnormal bounce can reveal clots in the thigh veins, and these clots are the origin of most pulmonary emboli. (Ultrasound won't pick up clots in the lungs because all the air gets in the way.)

A diagnostic ultrasound study, i.e., one showing clots in his thigh veins, would suggest the clots were about to break away; if that was the case, perhaps some clots had already traveled to his lungs and caused his chest pain and hemoptysis. This would be highly unusual given the normal lung scan, but I was fishing. True, he had no leg pain or swelling, but half the patients with leg clots have no symptoms. Finding clots in his legs would be sort of like diagnosing pulmonary emboli by proxy, especially since treatment is the same as for clots in the lungs.

But the ultrasound test was also normal. There were no clots in his legs, so we had to seek another reason for the pain and hemoptysis. The problem was that I could not think of another reason.

By now, Mr. McShane had been at Mt. Sinai Hospital over eight hours and it was late afternoon. I had no more tests planned for his first day of hospitalization. Before leaving, I went to see him again.

"So far, your tests are normal. They suggest you don't have pulmonary emboli. That's the good news."

"And the bad news, Doctor Martin?"

"Well, there really is no bad news, except that I don't know why you are coughing up blood again. You said they diagnosed pulmonary emboli last year in Atlanta?"

"Yes, that's right. My doctor was Dr. Howard Lee, Mercy Hospital. You saw his letter. My lung scan showed pulmonary emboli, and they were fairly certain of the diagnosis. Do you think it's cancer, Dr. Martin?"

"Cancer?" I said, with some surprise. I had not even been thinking of cancer to explain his symptoms. "No, I don't think it's cancer, not at your age. First, you don't smoke. Second, your chest x-ray is clear. Nothing to suggest cancer there. However, to be certain, I suppose I really should do a bronchoscopy. Sometimes cancer can cause hemoptysis and not be visible on the chest x-ray. I'd like to do the bronchoscopy tomorrow morning. I believe you had that procedure in Atlanta, right?"

"Yes, the first time I was hospitalized, not the second time. The first time is when they said the problem was just bronchitis. It's not the most pleasant test, but if you have to do it, I'm ready. Nothing to eat or drink after midnight, right?"

"Right." This guy certainly knew the protocol.

My beeper went off about a half hour later, as I was preparing to leave the hospital. It was Mr. McShane's nurse.

"Dr. Martin, can you come up? Mr. McShane just coughed up a whole lot of blood."

"OK. Please check his blood pressure and pulse, and put him on two liters of oxygen. I'll be right up."

My patient was sitting in his bed, holding a curved plastic basin full of blood. I estimated at least 30 cc's, or about two ounces, were in the basin. There was also a little bit of blood over his chin and lower lip. He appeared apprehensive, his face contorted in pain, and his pulse was rapid at 120/minute. A quick exam of his lungs and heart revealed nothing new.

"How do you feel? Do you have any chest pain?"

"Yes," he said quietly, with little complaint in his voice. "It came on just before the hemoptysis, all of a sudden. I'm sorry to bother you, Dr. Martin."

"Nonsense," I replied. "That's what we're here for. However, I think I should send you to the intensive care unit and do the bronchoscopy now, instead of tomorrow. I need to know the site of bleeding. You might end up requiring surgery, and for that we need to know where the blood is coming from. Does it feel like it's coming from your left lung? Can you tell?"

"I don't know...Doctor Martin. Maybe it's coming from both lungs... I just don't know. But the pain is severe, I can tell you that."

I ordered another injection of Demerol and set in motion his transfer to the ICU. I also paged one of the respiratory technicians, to help me set up the bronchoscope. With the supper time delay in transport, it took us another hour before Mr. McShane was settled in MICU and the bronchoscopy could start. By then, the Demerol had worked and he was calm. I also ordered injection of a sedative, to relax him for the bronchoscopy.

The bronchoscope allows physicians to look inside the lungs, much as gastroenterologists look into the stomach and intestines with an endoscope. Both techniques employ a thin fiberoptic device that is a marvel of engineering. The bronchoscope is much smaller than a gastrointestinal endoscope, only six mm wide (about 1/4 inch), two feet long and quite flexible (the formal term for the procedure is "flexible fiberoptic bronchoscopy").

We pass the bronchoscope through the mouth or nose and then into the lungs. Contained within the scope's six-mm diameter and running the entire length of the bronchoscope are: a narrow channel for suctioning mucous or blood from the patient's lungs; fiberoptic bundles for transmitting a bright light; other fiberoptic bundles that allow us to see through the scope; and a thin wire that allows us to bend the bronchoscope tip in almost any direction. By looking through the bronchoscope we can usually tell the site of bleeding as long as it has been recent, as Mr. McShane's episode was.

He was cooperative during the procedure. I passed the scope with no difficulty and was able to see all the major air passages in both lungs. But I saw no blood; it was all gone. This sometimes happens. The patient coughs up what little blood leaks into the air tubes, and by the time you get around to looking with the bronchoscope, the blood has disappeared, presumably all coughed out.

Well, he had surely had hemoptysis. I and the nurses saw the blood. Furthermore, he had a history of coughing up blood, and a diagnosis of pulmonary emboli was made in Atlanta. Then I began to wonder. Could the Atlanta doctors have been wrong about the diagnosis? Could they have missed another, more insidious cause, such as an uncommon autoimmune disease? Anything was possible, but given the findings to that point, I was still concerned about pulmonary embolism.

My plans were to watch him overnight and consider doing a pulmonary angiogram the next day, a test that, for all its faults, is considered the "gold standard" for diagnosing pulmonary emboli. One of the test's difficulties is that it is highly "invasive." A catheter has to be inserted into the heart's chambers so dye can be injected to outline blood vessels that serve the lungs. Clots show up nicely with this test, but the angiogram's invasiveness and expense limit its use. The lung scan is more indirect but much easier to perform. Perhaps only one out of every 100 patients initially suspected of having pulmonary embolism ends up with an angiogram.

That night, about ten p.m., I called the ICU to see how Mr. McShane was doing. No one had called me, so I knew he wasn't in shock or deteriorating, but I did have visions of him coughing up a little more blood and of the house staff fretting over when he might open up and exsanguinate. (We had typed his blood on admission and were prepared to transfuse if necessary). One of the MICU nurses answered the phone.

"Hi Greg, this is Dr. Martin, how's Mr. McShane doing?" Mr. McShane was only one of eight MICU patients that night and not the sickest by far, but he was the most recently admitted to the unit.

There was a short pause, then a slight, sardonic laugh. "Dr. Martin, he's just fine. No more hemoptysis. His heart's beating a little fast, but the rhythm's normal. The rest of his vital signs are stable." Greg didn't say it, of course, but his tone was unmistakable: 'What's this patient doing *here*? He seems to be too healthy for the intensive care unit.' But then Greg hadn't seen him upstairs, just before the ICU transfer.

"By the way, Dr. Martin, did you know this guy was once the United States welter weight boxing champion?"

"Really?" I know next to nothing about boxing, but Greg seemed impressed, and it was a facet of my patient new to me.

"Yea," Greg continued. "He was telling us how he won the title when he was only twenty-six, in Boston, but then he gave up fighting to join the U.S. merchant marines. This guy's been around."

"So he has," I said reflexively, not realizing how ironic my comment would soon seem. "Well, let's watch him overnight. You can transfer him if you need the bed for another patient. But call me if he coughs up any more blood."

* * *

Mr. McShane was transferred out of MICU early the next morning, to make space for another, far sicker patient. By the time I reached the hospital he was already back in his regular semi-private room. After checking the MICU patients, I went up to see him; it was about 8:30.

"I understand you've coughed up no more blood since the bronchoscopy. How are you feeling?"

"OK, I guess. That last injection helped quite a bit." I had left a standing Demerol order for severe pain. Since the bronchoscopy, he had received one more injection.

"Dr. Martin, are you going to do the angiogram this morning?"

"I'm not sure. I want to discuss that with you. So far, everything appears normal except for your fast heart rate, which I also cannot easily explain."

"Oh, I see. But if I don't have pulmonary embolism, what is causing my hemoptysis?"

"I don't know. And I can't treat you because I don't know what to treat for. Sometimes people cough up blood and we never find a cause. Then there is a group of autoimmune diseases that are difficult to diagnose, and they can cause hemoptysis. Some of the blood samples we drew yesterday are to check for these unusual diseases, and the results should be back later today.

"The one major procedure we haven't done is a pulmonary angiogram. This involves placing a long catheter into your heart and squirting some dye through it, to directly visualize any clots sitting in your lungs. It's an invasive test and probably unnecessary in your case, since your lung scan is normal. We usually recommend an angiogram when the lung scan is equivocal, but yours really isn't. In fact, in your situation the findings rule out pulmonary embolism with almost ninety-nine percent certainty. We'd need to do a pulmonary angiogram to make it one hundred percent, but I'm reluctant to push for an angiogram unless you understand these odds. Since it's an invasive test there are some risks, some potential complications."

I thought at the time: he *could* be one of those extremely rare individuals with a normal lung scan despite the pulmonary embolism. Faced with a strong story for embolism and a normal scan, some doctors would just watch him without doing any more tests or giving any treatment. The assumption, entirely valid, is that if a clot is present it is just too small to do any real harm. Other doctors might opt for doing the angiogram, on the theory that it is important to make a proper diagnosis and that maybe he should be treated even if the clot is only a small one.

It did not seem unreasonable to propose an angiogram, given the circumstances, and I was prepared to present my case. Mr. McShane was an intelligent patient with a serious problem, and he should be involved in the decision making. I expected a barrage of questions and further discussion leading up to an informed consent. To my surprise, he didn't hesitate.

"I understand everything you say, Dr. Martin. Let's do the angiogram. I want to know why I'm coughing up blood."

"Are you sure?"

"Yes."

"Don't you want to know the potential complications?"

"I trust you, Dr. Martin. If you recommend it, that's good enough for me."

I wanted informed consent, not "Yessir, anything you say, sir!" This guy was too eager. Too eager. No one has ever agreed so readily to have a pulmonary angiogram. Always, there are some questions, a quick consultation with the family, or some other hesitancy over having a catheter inserted into one's heart. I began to wonder (probably for the first time) about his psyche. He had a serious medical symptom but didn't seem to be handling it like a patient. What was the problem?

***

In retrospect, he was too smooth. I find this difficult to explain, but it seemed as if he was both the patient and *apart* from the patient. He had the proper symptoms but not the proper affect. Except when he complained of chest pain, I had the unsettling feeling he could put on a white coat and play *my* role, that of the detached professional. I needed to get out of his room and think things over.

"Okay," I said, "Let me see if I can set up the angiogram this morning. I'll be back to let you know soon."

I went to the nurse's station and for the next few minutes pondered the situation with his chart open in front of me. I wasn't exactly sure what to do next about making a diagnosis. There was a 99 percent chance a pulmonary angiogram would be normal. Should I subject him to this invasive procedure now, or do some other test, and if so, what test? Or just wait for results of the blood work which, at best, would be inconclusive? For a few minutes, my mind just wandered. Then it hit me, the logical next step.

I placed a call to the Atlanta hospital where he had been a patient the year before. A little more detail about his medical history couldn't hurt, and might even help decide what to do next. It was early, and I figured the physician might be making hospital rounds.

I made the call myself and had no trouble reaching the Atlanta hospital's switchboard operator. I introduced myself and asked if Dr. Howard Lee was in the hospital, and if not, could she please give me his office number. After the customary "One moment please," there was a long pause, perhaps half a minute.

"I'm sorry, Sir," she came back, "but we have no one here by that name. You did say Dr. Howard Lee?"

"Yes. Are you sure? Has he left the hospital staff?"

"I don't know, sir. I only have a list of active staff physicians. Are you sure you have the right hospital?"

A copy of the "To Whom It May Concern Letter" was in McShane's chart. I checked it again.

"Yes, I'm sure of that."

"Would you like me to connect you to the Office of Medical Staff? They would know if this doctor recently left the hospital."

"Yes, please."

I was connected to a secretary in Mercy's Medical Staff Office. She listened dutifully to my query, then put me on hold while she checked some records. She returned about two minutes later.

"I'm sorry to keep you waiting, Dr. Martin. We have no record of any such physician on our staff in the past five years. You say you have his letter on our hospital stationery?"

"Yes, right in front of me." I read her the heading, address and all. This bit of hard evidence intrigued her, as well it should.

"Would you mind faxing that letter to me? If you do that, I can show it to a few people and maybe help you that way."

My first thought was that this letter pertained to a patient of mine and that I could not send any part of the medical record without his permission. But this thought quickly dissipated as I contemplated the specific circumstances and how I came to have the letter in the first place.

"Yes, I'll fax it right now. Just do me a favor, please."

"What is that?"

"I need to make some decision about this patient fairly soon. Could you work on this now and get back to me by noon? Either way, even if you come up empty handed?"

"Yes, Dr. Martin. I'll do my best to find out more about this matter. And I'll get back to you either way."

"Thanks," I said and gave her my office and beeper numbers. It was now shortly after 9 a.m. I saw no reason to go back to Mr. McShane's room right away. I would wait until I had more information.

* * *

About 11 a.m. I was paged to the phone. It was Mercy Hospital's switchboard operator. She had a call for me from Dr. Howard Lucas, an Atlanta internist. I knew it was about McShane, but had no idea what to expect. What was the real story?

"Dr. Martin?"

"Yes."

"Hello. I'm Dr. Howard Lucas. Our medical affairs secretary faxed me your letter a few minutes ago, and asked me to call you. Hope I'm not interrupting something important." His voice was pleasantly southern, with long i's and soft consonants.

"No, Dr. Lucas, not at all. Thank you for calling. Maybe you can clear up a few things. Do you know about my patient or his letter? We admitted him to Mt. Sinai Hospital in Cleveland yesterday morning. He gave us the letter I sent. Said he was in your hospital for hemoptysis, and that Dr. Howard Lee took care of him. I gather there is no Howard Lee on your staff?"

Dr. Lucas let out a soft chuckle. "Yes, I'm afraid we know your patient. Beverly called the legal office when she got your fax. It seems that a patient checked out of here last year AMA [against medical advice], and before leaving, he had somehow managed to lift a bunch of hospital stationery and other supplies. And his name was Shane, John Shane. Well, I was his doctor, so Beverly called me next. Is your patient about five feet ten, slim, brown hair? Sort of looks athletic?"

"Yes, that's him. Then you had him in the hospital?"

"John Shane was our patient. Came in with hemoptysis, pretty convincing story. We did all sorts of tests but found nothing wrong. Yet he kept coughing up blood. He really had us puzzled. He had a lot of chest wall pain, too. Got Demerol about every six hours until we wised up.

181

"About his third or fourth day here, he coughed up blood while watching television in his room. He called a nurse over, and without taking his eyes off the screen said, "Here, here's some more blood," like he was giving her a urine sample or something. She thought his affect was strange, especially since she had been giving him injections for pain, and called me. By then we were mighty suspicious. I sent the "blood" for examination. Guess what? There was no blood in the sample! It was ketchup or something. The guy's a con artist. A real sicko. We're convinced he faked his hemoptysis the entire time. Sorry you got caught with him."

"Did you call in a psychiatrist?"

"Well, we were going to, but as soon as we exposed him, he signed out AMA. Haven't heard from or about him since. Until just now."

"Well, it certainly sounds like the same guy," I said. "He also told us he was in your hospital twice, about six months apart, and that the first time doctors just diagnosed bronchitis."

"Is that so? I'm sure we only had him once, the time I just told you about. I guess he makes up his story as he goes along."

"He also told us he's visiting his sister here. Said he's a computer salesman and lives in Atlanta with his family, a wife and two kids."

"Now that you mention it, I remember he told us he was from Texas or somewhere out west and was in Atlanta for an accountant's convention. I never heard about any family. I'm telling you, the guy's a looney tune. He sounds like a classic Munchausen. Didn't pay his bill, either. In fact, his insurance card was phony, and all his bills were returned with No Forwarding Address stamped on them. He stiffed the doctors and the hospital."

"I think I'm getting the picture. Thanks, Dr. Lucas. You've been very helpful."

"No problem. Glad to help. Good luck with this guy. See if you can get psychiatry to see him. He certainly needs their help."

I felt like someone had punched me in the stomach, deflated my tires, stolen my bicycle. What kind of person fakes a serious illness? And why? I went back to the room to confront Mr. McShane aka Shane. Although I now felt betrayed by this imposter, I had to remind myself he was still a patient and would remain so until I could confirm this bizarre story and transfer his care to a psychiatrist. So, in a quiet, non-confrontational manner, I walked back to his bedside. He spoke first.

"Did you arrange for the angiogram, Dr. Martin?"

"No, I called Mercy Hospital instead. In Atlanta."

He showed no concern, no surprise. After all, he had given me the hospital's name, so I guess he figured there was nothing to hide.

"I spoke with a Dr. Lucas. There is apparently no Dr. Howard Lee on their staff."

"Oh? Well, he must have left. But it was his letter, all right."

"Dr. Lucas says he took care of you last year, but that he knows you under a different name, as Mr. Shane, not *Mc*Shane."

"Sorry, doc, I changed it recently. Having some alimony problems. I should have told you."

Lucas not Lee. Shane not McShane. And sorry *doc*? What's this *doc*? For almost twenty-four hours it had been "Doctor Martin," formal, distancing. Now with his lies unraveling, I was being addressed *doc*, and spoken to with a touch of disdain. *Uh-oh.*

"He also said you claimed to be coughing up blood last year, but all they found under the microscope was ketchup, or something like ketchup."

I said these things calmly, matter-of-factly, careful not to sound like a prosecutor out to destroy the made-up alibi of some guilty defendant. My patient was sicker than anyone had realized, and an accusatory posture would not help the situation. He had to know we knew the truth and that we understood his needs were psychiatric, not medical. It would do no good to play his game, whatever that game was.

The truth was too much. At the mention of "ketchup" his head snapped into position and he stared straight at me. The intensity of his stare was frightening. If his eyes were lasers I am certain they would have burned two holes in my skull. After about ten seconds he spoke. There was anger in his voice.

"That is a bald... faced... LIE!"

The last word was yelled. I stepped back a pace, half expecting him to jump out of the bed and pummel me. Was he really an ex-welter weight?

He started to snarl, then contorted his face to express disgust: raised upper lip, flared nostrils, gritted teeth. Would he spit next? I decided to keep silent. The ball was in his court.

He relaxed his features. Then, with contempt in his voice: "Look, doc, you're a nice guy, but if YOU can't find the cause of my hemoptysis I'll go someplace else, to somebody COMPETENT. I don't need this phony accusation stuff thrown at me!"

A passing nurse entered the room, attracted by his loud voice. I motioned her to stay behind me, that everything was okay, and then tried to calm him down. I sensed my effort would be futile.

"I'm sorry, I'm just reporting what Dr. Lucas—"

"Lucas Schmucas," he interrupted. "He's a phony, too. Cut the crap, doc. Hey, whatever happened to your HIPPOCRATIC oath? Did you lose it somewhere? Maybe I can help you find it!"

Now he was visibly agitated. He jumped out of bed on the side opposite us and fidgeted with the night stand drawers. He opened a drawer and took out his clothes: pants, shirt ("blood"-stained), shoes and socks, and a folder full of papers (more letters?). In another two minutes he was out of his hospital gown and dressed in street clothes.

"Where are you going?"

"Sorry doc, you guys had your chance. Hey, what kind of doctor are you, anyway?"

"Mr. McShane, you need some help. Please stay and let us call a psychiatrist. You can't keep going from hospital to hospital with this complaint of hemoptysis. There's nothing wrong with your lungs. Somebody could do an unnecessary procedure and you could be harmed. Let us try to help you."

"Help me? Hah! You're the one who needs help. I've NEVER seen such unprofessional behavior. NEVER. And I've seen a lot, believe me!"

I kept my distance and did not reply. The nurse asked if she should call Security. No, I said, reminding myself that we can't keep patients against their will. Security would be no use in this situation.

In less than a minute our patient walked off the ward, took the elevator and was gone.

* * *

Con man? Not quite. A mentally ill man is more like it. Actually, Mr. Shane/McShane is a classic example of a condition long described in medical and psychiatric circles, the Munchausen Syndrome. The syndrome is named after an eighteenth-century German, popularly known as Baron von Munchausen, real name Karl Friedrich Hieronymus, Freiherr von Munchausen (1720-1797). Munchausen, a soldier who fought for the Russian Empire in the Russo-Turkish War of 1735–1739, was notorious for telling entertaining stories of outlandish proportion, entirely made up.

Munchausen's reputation was enlarged upon by a contemporary, one Rudolph Erich Raspe, who in 1785 anonymously published (in German) *Baron Munchausen's Narrative of His Marvellous Travels and Campaigns in Russia*. This work, a satire in that it included impossible feats performed by the Baron (riding a cannonball, fighting a forty-foot alligator, travelling to the moon), was soon translated into English as *The Adventures of Baron Munchausen.* The book became a popular work of the late eighteenth century and has since gone through many editions. It is currently available on in various editions, one of which is shown below, left.

The character and his stories have also been recreated for the stage, television and movies. The poster on right is from the 1988 film, which the critics praised (though it bombed at the box office).

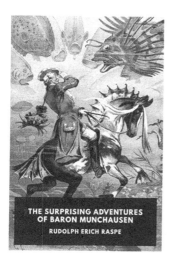 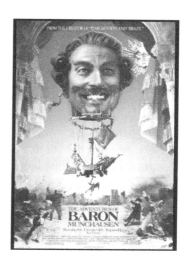

***

The term "Munchausen's Syndrome" was first used in a 1951 article in the British medical journal *The Lancet*. A group of patients repeatedly sought hospitalization by simulating symptoms of illness. Dr. Richard Asher, author of the article, wrote:

> Here is described a common syndrome which most doctors have seen, but about which little has been written. Like the famous Baron von Munchausen, the persons affected have always traveled widely; and their stories, like those attributed to him, are both dramatic and untruthful. Accordingly the syndrome is respectfully dedicated to the baron, and named after him.
>
> The patient showing the syndrome is admitted to hospital with apparent acute illness supported by a plausible and dramatic history. Usually his story is largely made up of falsehoods; he is found to have

> attended, and deceived, an astounding number of other hospitals; and he nearly always discharges himself against advice, after quarreling violently with both doctors and nurses...

Since the original article, there have been numerous medical reports of patients faking abdominal pain, seizures, kidney stones, back pain, asthma, mental confusion, fever, blood in the urine, hemoptysis, and a variety of other illnesses. Although Asher called the syndrome common, it may only appear common because one Munchausen patient may be seen by so many different physicians and at a variety of institutions. A review published in 1967 found only 59 cases reported in the literature to that time. Munchausen remains a rare syndrome. In the 1967 review Munchausen men outnumbered women three to one; the age range was 19-62 years, with a mean age of 39.

Typical features of the Munchausen patient include:

-- faking an acute illness that requires hospitalization
-- familiarity with medical terms and diseases
-- lack of any obvious external reason for seeking hospitalization
-- aggressive behavior toward health professionals when the truth of the symptoms is challenged
-- leaving the hospital against medical advice

Munchausen patients frequently travel from city to city, or even to several hospitals within one large metropolitan area. It is not unusual to uncover a string of hospital admissions within a one- or two-year period, and spanning several states. There is one report of a patient who had, over a 16-year period: 40 hospitalizations in three states for abdominal pain, chest pain, loss of consciousness, blood in the urine and fever, all apparently factitious; 32 emergency room visits for the same problems; four abdominal operations; and one brain operation. Whenever he presented to a hospital that had cared for him many times before, he always told the doctors it was his first time there.

Another patient, a 33-year-old man, was discussed in two separate articles in a single issue of the *New England Journal of Medicine* (August 6, 1992). The first article covered his evaluation for a puzzling disorder at Brooklyn's University Hospital in 1991. The second article discussed evaluation for the same disorder after he was admitted to Yale New Haven Hospital in early 1992. The problem? Sudden onset of coughing up *and* urinating blood. Doctors at Yale knew nothing about the previous evaluation in Brooklyn. At each hospital, after an extensive workup, his physicians diagnosed the Munchausen Syndrome and on both occasions the patient left AMA after he was exposed. The nature of his symptoms—coughing up *and* urinating blood—plus the ultimate diagnosis of Munchausen, led the Yale physician to title his report "The Red Baron."

Why do people fake a serious illness? No one knows for sure, but the problem is widely accepted as psychiatric in nature, a form of character disorder manifesting as antisocial behavior. Munchausen is not a psychosis like schizophrenia, and paradoxically is much harder to treat. These patients don't respond to tranquilizers or other mind-altering drugs.

Munchausen patients who have been studied by psychiatrists seem to have one thing in common: an unhappy, unloving childhood. Their early home life is often described as abusive and neglectful. As adults they become attention seeking, and in this way "act out" their rage over past deprivations. They seek nurturing for what they lacked in childhood.

Why does their nurture-seeking take place in hospitals? Because of some early experience, they have learned to manipulate the medical care system. A modicum of medical training is common. Tricking doctors and nurses seems to satisfy their need to get back at society, even if this behavior puts them at risk for harm (by having unnecessary tests and procedures).

The only effective treatment, if it can be called that, is to replace their episodic, and often chaotic, hospitalizations with intensive psychologic counseling in a chronic care facility, i.e., long-term care in a psychiatric institution. Suffice to say, it is the rare Munchausen who ends up in such an arrangement.

William Bean, an eminent physician of internal medicine, described one Munchausen patient in verse. His poem ended thus:

> I'm sorry I cannot fasten my claws on
> What causes the syndrome named Munchausen
> This off again, on again, gone again Finnegan
> Comes in, goes out, and at length comes in again.
> Munchausen's victims must be expected
> To plague our lives unless deflected.
> So be alert for this great nonesuchman
> Munchausen syndrome's flying Dutchman.
>
> William B. Bean, M.D. "The Munchausen Syndrome." *Perspectives in Biology and Medicine*, Spring 1959: 347-53.

* * *

Perhaps even more common than adult Munchausen Syndrome is the now well-described Munchausen by Proxy, where an adult, usually the mother, fakes a child's illness in order for the child to obtain medical attention. In this situation, there can be actual physical harm cause by the mother, or she may describe her child's symptoms that are either a gross exaggeration or outright fabrication.

Doctors aren't sure what causes Munchausen by Proxy, but it may be linked to problems during the abuser's childhood. Abusers often feel like their life is out of control. They often have poor self-esteem and can't deal with stress or anxiety. The attention that caregivers get from having a sick child may encourage their behavior. Caregivers may get attention not only from doctors and nurses but also from others in their community. For example, neighbors may try to help the family in many ways, such as by doing chores, bringing meals, or giving money.

One of the worst cases of Munchausen by Proxy was made into a 2017 HBO documentary, *Mommy Dead and Dearest*. The mommy, Dee Dee Blanchard, was the perpetrator, and through fake illness after fake illness, turned her daughter, Gypsy Rose, into a wheelchair-bound invalid. In the end, Gypsy Rose conspired with her boyfriend to have her mother killed. In 2016, at age twenty-four, Gypsy Rose was sentenced to ten years in prison for second-degree murder.

***

Several puzzling questions remain about Mr. Shane/McShane. What caused his fast pulse? The heart beats involuntarily. Unless you exercise or take a stimulant, you can't accelerate the rhythm. Likely he took some stimulant to keep his heart beating fast and make us think he had a serious medical problem. Except for this abnormality, he was the picture of health, and should have had a normal or even slow heart beat (like a true athlete). We never found the stimulant, but then we didn't have a chance to look. Had he stayed around we would have ordered a blood test for various stimulants.

Why did he make up a history that was easy to verify as false? This feature is sometimes seen in Munchausen patients when the previous medical care has been in another state. Sometimes they carry medical records with them, conveniently doctored or, as in this case, wholly fabricated on stolen stationery. They probably think physicians won't check out the story in any detail.

Munchausen patients are good at faking medical symptoms and complaints. These symptoms rivet the doctor's attention, so that details about career and travels are seldom an initial concern and not something we try to verify—until our suspicions are raised, of course. I am sure his background was also fabricated, that he was not a computer salesman or, for that matter, an ex-boxer or accountant. His slight name change from what he called himself in Atlanta may represent some private conceit; perhaps it allowed him to believe he was covering his trail, so to speak, while at the same time keep the story straight in his own mind.

Where did the blood come from? We never knew, but then we never analyzed the material he coughed up. Hemoptysis is relatively common and Munchausen Syndrome is very rare, so when someone coughs up red mucous we don't ask, "Is he faking it? Is this really blood?" Most likely, Mr. McShane kept a supply of fake blood in his clothes and produced it at will. Probably not ketchup, per se, but the same stuff used in the movies to simulate bleeding.

Finally, where did he go? In typical Munchausen fashion, he likely went to other hospitals and fooled other doctors. As expected, the number he gave for his "sister" drew a "not-in-service" response. The insurance information he provided the hospital was phony, and his medical bills went unpaid.

– END –

20. "Mommy, why don't you hug me?"

Thirty-five-year-old Naomi Benedict was sitting in a chair at home, recovering from the flu, when she felt a sudden tingling in both legs. She stood up to stretch, lost her balance and promptly fell to the floor.

The maid ran in from the kitchen. What was wrong? Mrs. Benedict said the only problem was her legs. They felt weak and tingly, as if their circulation was cut off. Otherwise she felt fine. The maid helped her stand up, then climb the stairs to the bedroom and get into bed.

It was two in the afternoon on Tuesday, March 7. Mr. Benedict, an attorney, was at work and their two young children were in school. At three o'clock she was to attend the city's Arts Council meeting, her first time out in a week. Instead of getting dressed, she lay in bed, unsure what to do.

She called her husband. Julian Benedict thought her leg weakness was probably from the flu and sitting too long in one position. He suggested she call Dr. Cooper and not try to make the meeting.

Dr. Cooper, one of the town's leading internists, knew the Benedicts well as both their physician and friend. He advised her to stay in bed; if not substantially better in the morning, after a good night's sleep, she should come to his office.

The next morning I was in the medical ICU making rounds, when Dr. Cooper phoned.

"Larry, I've got Naomi Benedict in my office. You know who she is, don't you?"

"Sure," I said, "her husband is Julian Benedict, right? I've seen their picture in the magazines." I did not know them personally, but I knew *of* them. At the time he was a rising young lawyer, famous after his defense of a business tycoon charged with murder. When his client won acquittal Julian Benedict's name was all over the papers. At age thirty-nine, he was a legal star.

I was aware of Naomi as a young socialite and heiress to a family fortune made in the steel industry. Like many young and wealthy women, she was active in prominent charities, one of which made donations to Mt. Sinai Hospital. She and her husband were also well known, at least locally, because of their home. "La Maison Magnifique,," so dubbed by an overly enthusiastic editor, was featured in the city magazine four months earlier. The Benedicts had spent a fortune redecorating an old French chateau-style mansion into something that, even by European standards, was stunning, at least from the magazine pictures (I have never been inside). Naomi's college degree was in art history and she had orchestrated the entire project.

"Well, I've been treating her for a viral gastroenteritis the past week," Dr. Cooper continued. "She had the flu with some diarrhea and was getting better, at least until yesterday. She had a little leg weakness yesterday and this morning can hardly walk. I'm not sure, but it might be progressive. She also has some diminished breath sounds. I did a vital capacity [a measure of lung function] in the office, and it's down to about seventy percent of predicted. Larry, I'm worried about her. I'd like to put her in MICU if you have a bed."

Dr. Cooper is known for good medical judgment, so if he worries about a patient, I do too. "Of course," I said. "We'll get a bed ready for her. When do you think she'll be here?"

"Well, Julian's with her, and he'll bring her down to the hospital. With her difficulty walking, it'll take them about half an hour."

"OK. We'll be ready."

A few minutes later Grayson McAllister, Mt. Sinai's Director of Neurology, stopped by. Just past forty, tall and aristocratic in bearing, Grayson is a neurologist's neurologist, which is to say he regularly consults on the rich and famous. Even in the era of CAT and magnetic resonance scanners, neurologic diagnosis is an art based on thorough history and detailed physical examination. Dr. McAllister is an artist.

"Hello, Grayson, what's up? Who are you here to see?"

"No one just yet. I understand Naomi Benedict is being admitted soon."

"Yes, that's right. Did Dr. Cooper call you also?"

"He left a message with my secretary to see her right away. When do you expect her?"

"Within the hour. I just talked to Cooper a few minutes ago."

"OK. Would you please page me as soon as she arrives?"

"Sure."

A few minutes later the Chief of the Department of Medicine walked in. He pulled me aside from rounds, to speak privately.

"Larry, Naomi Benedict is being admitted to your MICU. She apparently has—"

"I know," I interrupted, somewhat surprised by this unexpected visit from my boss. "I spoke with Dr. Cooper a while ago, and Grayson McAllister was just here also."

"Well, I just came to tell you about Julian, her husband. I don't think you know him. He's on the hospital's board of trustees. He's one of the nicest guys you'll ever meet, a tiger in court, but outside the courtroom he's a real gentleman. Naomi works on the hospital's auxiliary. I can't tell you how much money she's helped raise for Mt. Sinai. I know them both. Don't be intimidated by their wealth or position. They are down-to-earth people. She, especially, is a doll. I sure hope she's okay. Maybe Dr. Cooper is just being over-cautious. Anyway, call me if you need assistance of any kind. We want to do everything necessary to help her."

I wanted to reply that "everything necessary" is what we do for all our patients, but instead just thanked the chief for his well-intentioned advice. Some degree of anxiety is natural when VIPs (or their relatives) become patients. Socially prominent people, including politicians, business leaders, and movie stars, always expect (and usually receive) special treatment. The difference is in nuances of service, not in basic medical care. In fact, doctors sometimes have to be careful not to let "VIP care" affect sound medical practice.

A desire not to intrude, not to bother, can actually inhibit physicians from doing an important test or procedure, although this is less likely to happen in MICU. I learned long ago that all patients, whether dope addict or corporation president, or the rich wife of a hot shot trial lawyer, want, and deserve the same thing: good medical care delivered in a friendly and compassionate manner.

A few minutes later, the swinging doors to MICU opened and an attendant ushered in Mrs. Benedict in a wheel chair. Julian Benedict walked beside her. From TV and magazine photos, I recognized them right away, although Julian appeared shorter than I had imagined. A three-piece business suit covered his stocky, muscular frame. Clean-shaven, tie perfectly knotted, he appeared ready to go to court. Naomi, also smartly dressed in street clothes, carried a purse on her lap.

Unlike most patients admitted to MICU, she was fully alert and in no distress. My first thought was that perhaps she didn't need to be in MICU, that she might be more comfortable in a private room in one of the hospital towers. My second thought was that the towers are not equipped to closely monitor patients, and if Dr. Cooper wanted close observation, she probably should be in MICU.

The MICU nurses went right to work. Since the Benedicts had bypassed normal admission procedures, they sent Mr. Benedict to the admitting office to provide insurance information and sign some papers. Then they took Mrs. Benedict into ICU Room 2 and exchanged her street clothes for a hospital gown. After a few minutes, Emily, one of the RN's, came out to get a bed scale. She gave me a knowing smile.

"Why the look?" I asked.

"Anne Klein skirt and blouse? Gucci shoes and purse? Can you believe it?"

I acted dumb. "Is that fancy?"

A rhetorical question, at least for Emily. She changed her expression to show that I was quite out of touch and returned to Mrs. Benedict's room.

Since Mrs. Benedict could not stand up, the nurses measured her height lying supine as five feet five inches. Next, they recorded temperature (normal), blood pressure (125/72), heart rate (105 beats per minute), respiratory rate (18 breaths a minute, normal), and skin turgor (normal). They hoisted her on a stretcher over the bed to obtain her weight (129 pounds), and attached EKG monitor leads to her chest. From that moment her heart rate and rhythm were continuously displayed on a bedside monitor.

When the nurses finished, I put in a page for Dr. McAllister and, accompanied by Janice Dover, one of the MICU interns, went in to see our new patient. Even without the fancy clothes, she was so different from our usual intensive care patient (elderly or debilitated or acutely ill). Here in MICU was a very attractive woman: light complexion, brown hair combed straight back, little makeup, with the poise and bearing of a top fashion model. Even in the bare cloth of a hospital gown, without jewelry, she looked elegant, a word never before associated with an arriving inpatient.

"Mrs. Benedict, I'm Dr. Martin and this is Dr. Dover. I supervise the ICU, and Dr. Dover is one of our interns. Dr. Cooper called when you were in his office, and told me something of your problem."

She smiled, then spoke with a mixture of embarrassment and concern. "Hello. I feel so foolish being here. Do you really think the intensive care unit is necessary? I don't feel sick."

"Well, Dr. Cooper is worried about your sudden weakness."

"I know. I just can't walk. I feel so helpless. What do you think it is?"

"We don't know yet. He wants us to watch you for a day or so and run some tests. If there is no progression of the weakness, you'll go home or to another part of the hospital to recuperate. He's also asked the head of our Neurology division to see you. That's Dr. McAllister. He will be down in a few minutes."

"Can my husband come in for just a minute? I want to tell him not to wait around. It's not necessary."

I checked her vital signs from the nurse's records. They were all normal except for the slightly fast heart rate. "Sure, I'll see if he's through in the admitting office."

Julian returned to MICU and went in to see his wife. He came out five minutes later and announced he was leaving the hospital for a few hours. She had insisted he go to work and come back in the afternoon, when more would be known about her condition. There would be no problem with their two children, since the Benedicts had a full-time housekeeper.

About this time, Dr. McAllister returned to MICU. Consultants on new admissions don't usually appear until after the intern has examined the patient, but in this case Dr. McAllister was asked to get involved right away. He apologized for "intruding" so soon and suggested we interview her together, then let him do the neurologic exam. This approach was reasonable since it would obviate repetition of her medical history.

Dr. McAllister introduced himself and began eliciting her story, the outline of which is related above. Mrs. Benedict had no trouble speaking or recalling events leading up to hospitalization. She impressed us as bright and articulate and, for all the press hype, remarkably free of affectation, an ordinary (if rich) human being who wanted nothing more than to get better and go home. On a personal level, I felt sorry for her.

Accustomed to all the druggies, alcoholics, and non-compliant patients we routinely see, as well as those in coma or serious distress, her presence in MICU seemed anomalous. She wasn't even sick. I couldn't get the idea out of my head: what is she *doing* here? Her weakness could progress, but in the scheme of things, why should it? She hadn't done anything "bad" to justify a serious illness. No drugs, no alcohol, no promiscuity.

But of course, these were foolish thoughts. There are many more diseases than those brought on by self-abuse. I reflected on Eric Siegel's *Love Story* and its depressing ending: innocence and happiness dashed by cruel fate. Mrs. Benedict was innocent. She had caught a virus and developed muscle weakness. Now, she could crash just like any other patient with a bad disease.

Another question from Dr. McAllister interrupted my ruminations. "Mrs. Benedict, did you run a fever when you had the flu?"

"I took my temperature only twice. Once, at the beginning of the flu, it was a hundred and one. Two or three days later it was down to one hundred. I haven't taken it since, but think I'm recovered from the flu. At least I feel better."

"Before you developed leg weakness, that is, before yesterday, did you have any numbness or tingling of your arms or legs?"

"No. The weakness and tingly feeling came on at the same time."

"Have the numbness and tingling persisted?"

"Yes. My legs have a tingling feeling now, like they're still asleep."

"But you have sensation in your legs? You can feel the bed sheets?"

"Yes, but my legs feel almost like they're not part of me, like they're still asleep."

"Have you had any trouble breathing?"

"No. Well, wait a minute. Yesterday I did feel a little short of breath after climbing the stairs. And this morning, getting into the car, I guess I was a little winded, but that's all. It's probably because I feel so tired."

"Do you smoke?"

"No, not at all."

"How about your husband?"

"Smoke? No, Julian doesn't smoke either."

"Have you ever had any respiratory problems, pneumonia, asthma, any lung trouble before?"

"No, nothing. This is actually the first time I've been in the hospital since Kevin, our youngest, was born. That was six years ago. In fact, I felt great until last week."

"Do you do any regular exercise?"

"Yes! Doubles tennis. Twice a week."

"When was the last time you played?"

"Two weeks ago. I haven't played since I got the flu."

"There was no fall-off in your game? I mean, the last time you played, did everything seem normal in your game?"

Here she gave a little laugh. "Yes. I mean, we lost, but I felt fine."

"Other than the weakness in your legs, have you noticed weakness anywhere else?"

She opened and closed her fists a few times. "No, I feel fine everywhere else."

"Has your weakness increased since yesterday? Is it harder for you to walk this morning than when you first noticed the weakness?"

"Yes. Yesterday, even after I fell on the floor, I could walk a little. This morning, my legs were weaker. Julian had to practically carry me into and out of the car. I could not make it by myself. Now I couldn't walk if I had to."

"Have you had any problem with your period? Is it regular?"

"Yes."

"Any history of kidney or heart disease?"

"No, none."

"How about arthritis?"

"No."

"Do you take any medication?"

"No, only what Dr. Cooper prescribed last week."

"What was that?"

"Erythromycin [an antibiotic] and some Donnatal [an anti-spasmodic for the diarrhea]."

"You've taken no other drugs the past few months?"

"Oh, an occasional aspirin. But nothing else."

"Have you eaten anything rotten or that tasted rotten in the past few weeks?"

"No. Nothing. Do you think this could be food poisoning?"

"Probably not. Botulism—and I *don't* think you have botulism—can sometimes present with progressive weakness."

There were several more questions about possible exposure to insect spray, toxic chemicals, and other people with similar afflictions, but the answers were all negative. In essence, her history was straightforward: a healthy and active woman; flu-like illness for about a week; development of abrupt leg weakness; progression over the ensuing 18 hours.

Next came the neurologic exam. Dr. McAllister was a marvel to watch as he tested her sense of smell and taste, eye movements in all directions, strength of muscles from neck to toes, reflexes, and numerous other aspects of nerve function. His exam was meticulous, thorough, and kind. He explained any poke or prod that might cause some discomfort.

Apart from findings in her lower extremities, the neurologic exam was "unremarkable." Her legs revealed the problem. Normally we can push our toes down (a motion called 'dorsiflexion') with great strength, as when pushing against a bed board or standing on our tip toes; Mrs. Benedict could not push down at all. While lying flat, we can lift our legs into the air and hold them up for at least a few seconds. She could not lift her legs even a fraction of an inch. We can easily take one leg and cross it over the other, from knee to ankle. This, too, she could not do. All she could accomplish with either leg was a slight rolling motion on the bed sheet.

She had sensation in both legs and could feel Dr. McAllister's warm hands and the gentle prick of his safety pin. Also of diagnostic importance was the *absence* of muscle reflexes in her legs. Normally, there is a reflex jerking of the leg if the knee is tapped with a rubber hammer. Her legs didn't budge.

After the history and exam, which took about an hour, we thanked her and went to the nurses' station.

"What do you think?" Dr. McAllister asked Dr. Dover.

"Well, she can't dorsiflex [push down] her feet, so there's weakness there.

It looks like a primary motor weakness of the lower extremities."

"Exactly," he commented. "And coming on a week after a viral illness, it makes you think of one particular diagnosis."

"Guillain-Barré syndrome?"

"Very good, Dr. Dover! Yes, she has the classic picture of Guillain Barré syndrome. The weakness began in her feet and seems to be progressing upwards. Now her thigh muscles are weak. I'm also a little worried about her breathing. Larry, I didn't detect any respiratory muscle weakness but that can happen if this progresses any further. We should check her vital capacity several times a day. Until we see which way she's going, I definitely want her to stay here. In the meantime, we'll need to do an LP [lumbar puncture] and an EMG [electromyogram] to help secure the diagnosis."

* * *

Georges Guillain and Jean A. Barré, two early twentiety-century French neurologists, were among the first to describe inflammation of the peripheral nerves leading to paralysis. They recognized that the paralysis occurred most commonly after a respiratory infection. Today the eponym "Guillain-Barré" is widely used for the syndrome of post-infection paralysis.

In GBS, myelin sheaths covering the motor nerves are damaged, and the nerves so affected don't transmit impulses. An analogy is the rubber sheath around a thin piece of metal wire that, when damaged, may prevent the wire from transmitting electricity. The specific cause of nerve sheath damage is unknown, though it is probably related to antibodies generated by the infectious agent (usually a virus).

GBS afflicts men more than women and can strike at any age. The most benign cases show only minor muscle weakness and then remit altogether. The most severe cases go on to total paralysis. If the myelin sheaths regenerate (which happens most of the time), and the patient doesn't die from acute respiratory or cardiac failure, the prognosis for recovery is good. Joseph Heller, the celebrated author of *Catch-22*, developed severe paralysis from GBS and recovered.

GBS classically presents as *ascending paralysis*, meaning it starts in the legs and progresses up the body. Atypically, paralysis can start in the head (with facial and eye muscle weakness, for example) and *descend* or start in the middle of the body (arm weakness) and travel both ways. The worst fear is paralysis of the respiratory or breathing muscles.

To have some idea what this type of respiratory failure is like do the following. Stop breathing without holding your breath. Instead, keep your mouth and throat open but do not move your chest (rib) cage. Keep your chest perfectly still. When you can no longer do so, notice how much your chest cage moves as you take in the very next breath. If you couldn't move your chest you would asphyxiate—in about four minutes.

A totally paralyzed patient cannot breathe because her chest cage doesn't move. Without movement, there is no expansion of the lungs, and without expansion no fresh air can enter the blood. All totally paralyzed patients require artificial ventilation for as long as the paralysis lasts.

Examination of the spinal canal fluid, the clear liquid that bathes the spinal cord, can help secure the diagnosis of GBS. Spinal fluid is removed for analysis through a hollow needle inserted in the middle of the back, at the level of the hips; the procedure is called a "spinal tap."

Reach around your back to the spine just between your hips. With the tips of your fingers feel the protuberances of the spinal column. In a spinal tap the needle goes between these two protuberances. A few drops of spinal fluid are removed and sent to the lab for analysis of protein, glucose, and cell count. A spinal tap is technically not difficult and is often done by house staff.

* * *

"I better do the spinal tap," said Dr. McAllister, "but it doesn't have to be done right away. Why don't you finish your workup, then call me? By the way, I met Mr. Benedict on his way out. I'll talk to him again when he comes back this afternoon."

Dr. Dover and I returned to finish the physical exam, since Dr. McAllister did not dwell on her heart, lungs or abdomen. Apart from the neurologic system, everything was normal. We also drew blood for routine tests and did the vital capacity measurement. Our exam and tests took about 45 minutes.

Afterwards, I paged Dr. McAllister. He returned to MICU and obtained permission from Mrs. Benedict for the spinal tap. The major complication, he explained, was "post-spinal-tap" headache, which occurs in perhaps fifteen percent of patients.

While she lay on one side, he injected a local anesthetic into a small area of skin over her spinal column. In a few minutes the area was fully numb. He then inserted an eighteen-gauge spinal needle into the space between two vertebral bodies. The needle entered her spinal canal with a slight "give." Success. Out flowed crystal-clear spinal fluid. One. . . two. . . three. . . four cc's. The precious fluid was collected and the needle withdrawn. Mrs. Benedict reported no pain from the procedure.

"I'll check the lab results," he said, "and call Dr. Cooper to let him know how she's doing. In the meantime, please page me when Mr. Benedict arrives. By the way, were you able to get the vital capacity?"

"Yes. It's slightly low," I said. "Three point two liters. We also did an arterial blood gas, which is normal."

In four hours, we had accomplished a battery of tests and exams that would have taken much longer on the general medical ward. We had also made a tentative diagnosis and plan of action, and set up a chart of items to follow her course: muscle strength of upper and lower extremities; vital capacity; respiratory rate; body temperature; blood pressure; and heart rate.

Those first few hours convinced me she was in the right place. Ascending paralysis can move fast. Doctors and nurses have to be prepared to move faster.

* * *

She went rapidly downhill. By four p.m., slightly over 24 hours after the onset of leg weakness and six hours after arriving in MICU, she began losing strength in her arms. More ominous, her respiratory rate increased to 28 breaths per minute and vital capacity fell to 2.1 liters. I met with Dr. McAllister.

"What do you think?" I asked.

"She's progressing, no doubt about it," he said. "I'm going to start plasmapheresis right away."

"Can that reverse such a rapid slide?"

"Sometimes yes, sometimes no. It's best if plasmapheresis is started before the patient ends up on a ventilator. The sooner the better. There was a large-scale study a few years ago on plasmapheresis in GBS. Something like 250 patients. They found definite improvement in patients who received plasmapheresis. But you have to start it early in the course."

"Aren't you surprised by how fast she's progressing?"

"Yes, I am. GBS usually progresses over a few days or weeks, rarely over a few hours. I've seen one other patient progress this fast. And there are some cases like this in the literature. Dr. Cooper sure knew what he was doing by putting her in MICU."

Dr. McAllister called the plasmapheresis service. The physician in charge agreed with the plan and arranged for technicians to begin pheresis that same evening.

They didn't get a chance. As Dr. McAllister was hanging up the phone an alarm went off in Mrs. Benedict's room. We ran in. Her pulse was 160 and she was *very short of breath.*

"Dr. Martin!" she gasped.

I was shocked by the change. Neck muscles contracted with each breath, and her skin was mottled and blue. Her speech was short, interrupted, gasping.

"What's..... the matter?..... What's happening to me?........ Why can't

I......breathe?"

Paralysis had ascended so rapidly that her diaphragm, the major breathing muscle that sits between the abdomen and chest, was now totally paralyzed. She was breathing only with "backup" neck muscles, and those were about to fail.

I spoke quickly to the nurse. "Please hand me the Ambu bag. And call anesthesia. She needs to be intubated right away." I began manual Ambu ventilation with 100 percent oxygen through a tight-fitting face mask. This would keep her breathing until we could get her intubated.

"Just breathe through this mask, Mrs. Benedict. You'll be fine," I reassured her.

Patients who can't breathe because of *lung* disease usually flail their arms and move their chest cage rapidly in and out. Mrs. Benedict did not have lung failure; her lungs, the organs of respiration inside the chest cage, were normal. Her respiratory muscles had failed, and she could not expand her chest. There was *no* movement of her chest, except when some air was pushed in by my squeezing the Ambu bag. Without artificial breathing assistance she would die.

The anesthesiologist came right away and intubated her with a foot-long, one-third-inch-wide plastic tube; one end of the tube stuck out from her mouth, and the other end disappeared into her throat. With the tube in place we had a secure airway, and as soon as we connected the tube to the ventilator she "pinked up." The ventilator, replete with alarms and frequently checked by respiratory therapists, was now her life support.

A quick physical exam uncovered no permanent damage. Blood pressure, heart rate, and skin perfusion were all reasonable. But what a close call! My patient almost died and, what's more, I felt certain *she* knew it.

I checked an arterial blood gas, which was adequate, then called Dr. Cooper and Mr. Benedict. Both men said the same thing: "I'll be right down."

* * *

Julian went in to visit his wife. I also went in the room, mainly to observe the cardiac monitor in case there was an autonomic surge. Despite modest sedation, Naomi's mind was completely intact. The distress of being fully aware yet unable to speak or move could lead to tachycardia.

"Naomi, this is Julian. Can you hear me?"

For the moment she lay there, motionless, eyes closed, a beautiful woman with a tube in her throat, surrounded by machines and monitors and wires.

"Julian, give her a gentle nudge," I said.

He touched her shoulder. "Naomi, this is Julian. Can you hear me?"

She opened her eyes and nodded her head, slowly.

"Hi, honey. The kids send their love. I told them you're doing fine. It's five o'clock now. They're home with Gertrude, eating supper."

Tears came to her eyes.

"We miss you, honey. You'll be home soon. The doctors say this paralysis is a short-term thing, that it's completely reversible. Do you understand what I'm saying?"

More tears. And in Julian's eyes, too. I wiped Naomi's tears away with a towel. It was an awkward moment, and I wanted to leave them alone. Her heart rhythm looked stable on the monitor, so I left the room. Julian emerged about ten minutes later, his face freshly washed. Neither of us said a word.

Just then, Dr. McAllister appeared. The three of us went into a MICU conference room, a small, square space almost completely filled with a round wood table. I hastily moved books and journals off the table. We sat down and I led off the discussion.

"Obviously, her condition has progressed, much faster than anyone expected. Unfortunately, one of the worst things has happened. The paralysis has affected her breathing muscles. She is stable but right now can't breathe without the ventilator. We plan to start a treatment called plasmapheresis, to wash out antibodies from her blood."

"What's that?" Julian asked quickly.

Dr. McAllister answered. "As Dr. Martin said, it's a technique that removes plasma and gets rid of antibodies that might be damaging her nerves. We think antibodies against the nerves are responsible for destroying the myelin sheaths or nerve coverings. We wash out the antibodies with a series of plasma exchanges over two weeks, five or six treatments total. It's fairly safe, and there are relatively few complications."

"Does she have to receive blood transfusions with this?"

"No, not at all. We infuse albumin to replace the plasma that's removed. There's no risk of AIDS or hepatitis, if that's what you're concerned about."

"And you say two weeks?"

"Yes. That's the standard length of time most patients are treated. We probably won't see much improvement before two weeks, either."

Mr. Benedict did not react to this information. Instead, he looked at me. "Dr. Martin, you said 'one of the worst' things. What's the worst?"

"Well, people can die from Guillain-Barré syndrome. I think you know that. It usually happens not from the paralysis itself, because we can support her breathing indefinitely, but from what we call autonomic dysfunction. The autonomic part of the nervous system controls things like heart rate and blood pressure. We don't understand why, but sometimes people with this condition can have a sudden surge of adrenalin. This can cause severe blood pressure swings and cardiac arrhythmia. If there is no autonomic crisis, and her nerve coverings regenerate as they usually do, she can fully recover. That's what we're aiming for, of course."

Mr. Benedict addressed Dr. McAllister. "I know her breathing is impaired, but is there any sign of recovery in the rest of her body?"

"No, but that's not surprising. It's usually progressive paralysis and then recovery, rather than some areas getting better while others get worse. Right now, I'd say she's nowhere near the recovery phase. We probably won't see any significant improvement for a week or more, even with plasmapheresis."

"I understand," he said. "Well, the kids want to see their mom. I told them they can't see her now because she has a bad infection and they might catch it. I really don't want them to see her like this, but if she improves, can they visit her here?"

"Sure," I said, "but I agree now's not the time. It would be much better when she's more awake and can interact with them. In fact, if there is no dramatic improvement in the next two days, I'm going to recommend a tracheostomy. That will allow us to take the endotracheal tube out of her mouth and put it through a small hole in her neck. Then she can eat, smile, and stay on the ventilator as long as necessary."

"She might not be able to eat just yet," interjected Dr. McAllister. "Sometimes this condition can affect the swallowing muscles. I wouldn't be surprised if hers are already involved, the way this thing has progressed."

He was right, of course. I should have thought of swallowing difficulty before saying she could eat with the tracheostomy. "That's true," I agreed. "But I would still recommend a tracheostomy for reasons of comfort."

"Well," replied Mr. Benedict, "let's cross that bridge when we come to it."

Plasmapheresis was started that evening. There was no immediate response, but none was expected so soon, and she remained ventilator-dependent. In fact, her paralysis progressed and by the next morning she could not move even her head. Only her eyes moved. We took advantage of this last vestige of motor function to teach her to answer "yes" (eyes up and down) and "no" (side to side). Dr. Dover inserted a thin stomach tube through her nose to be used for feedings. Other tubes already inserted included large intravenous lines for the plasmapheresis and a bladder catheter for collecting urine.

There was no change in her condition after 48 hours. I called Mr. Benedict about the need for tracheostomy, and he gave permission. The operation was done on Thursday afternoon by a surgeon. She returned from the operating room with the tracheostomy tube in place and her face free of any encumbrance except for the small feeding tube in one nostril.

By the end of the third day we had results of several tests, all of which were consistent with GBS. The spinal fluid protein was slightly elevated. Since the protein content reaches a peak value several days into the illness, Dr. McAllister thought the small rise merely reflected an early measurement. An EEG or electroencephalogram, done the day after she "crashed," was normal except for some mild sedative effect, also consistent with GBS. The EEG tests brain wave activity and not peripheral nerves impulses, as does the EMG. Her EMG showed normal muscles but abnormal nerve conduction within the muscles, an impairment typically seen in GBS.

* * *

On the evening of the third day, about one hour after her second plasmapheresis, the nurses turned her to change the bed sheets. Almost immediately Mrs. Benedict's heart rate increased from 95 to 160, and blood pressure bottomed out at 65/30. The nurses quickly rolled her back and pushed a button to lower the head of the bed to the Trendelenburg position, (named after the German surgeon Friedrick Trendelenburg). In this position the body is angled about 30 degrees with the head down, to facilitate blood flow to the brain.

The MICU resident reacted swiftly to the autonomic crisis. She ordered a "wide open" saline infusion and intravenous verapamil, a drug that can slow a too-rapidly-beating heart. These measures worked, and in five minutes her blood pressure was up to 110/64 and heart rate down to 112. I was not in MICU at the time, but it didn't matter; I could not have done a better job. For the next few days the nurses were advised to turn Mrs. Benedict very slowly and with an eye on the monitor.

On Saturday, March 11, Dr. McAllister and I met again with Mr. Benedict. "As you can see, she's doing about the same," I said. "Since last night's episode of low blood pressure she's been quite stable. She still needs the ventilator and will probably stay on it for some time."

"We're going to continue the plasmapheresis another week to ten days," added Dr. McAllister. "By then we should see some improvement, although I must tell you I have seen paralysis continue for months before there is significant nerve sheath regeneration."

Julian listened intently, then spoke. This time it was he who had something to tell us. "A member of my firm did some work for one of the New York hospitals. He made some inquiries when I told him about Naomi's condition and obtained the name of a neurologist there. I hope you two don't mind if this doctor consults on Naomi."

"Not at all, not at all," said Dr. McAllister, mildly surprised.

"It's certainly OK with me," I added.

"Who is it?" asked Dr. McAllister.

"Dr. Byron DeJong."

At this, Dr. McAllister raised his eyebrows. "Well, you certainly picked a winner. He's probably the world's top authority on GBS. I've heard him speak several times."

"Good. I didn't know you knew him, but I'm glad you have no objection. I trust you guys implicitly. I wouldn't be on the board if I didn't think this is a damn good hospital. I have to do this for myself. If for some reason Naomi doesn't make it, I want to know I did everything possible."

"I understand perfectly," said Dr. McAllister. "When's he coming in?"

"Tomorrow. He could only come on Sunday. I'm picking him up at the airport tomorrow morning."

* * *

That afternoon I went to the library and read most of Dr. DeJong's recent papers on Guillain-Barré syndrome. Although our specialties were different, I didn't want to seem ignorant of his work. His publications were mostly clinical, dealing with natural history of the disease, effect of various treatments, and long term follow-up of patients. In these areas, he was an authority on GBS.

There was no change in Mrs. Benedict's condition all day Saturday. On Sunday, Mr. Benedict and his New York consultant showed up in MICU about 11 a.m. Dr. DeJong, about 50 years old, was dressed casually: a sport coat without tie, denim trousers, and comfortable loafers. His personality seem to match: low key, self-assured, friendly. The only thing he brought to the ICU was a large briefcase full of neurologic testing equipment. I wondered what he was charging for this out-of-town visit, on what was most likely his day off. Whatever the fee, it probably didn't matter to Mr. Benedict.

I handed him Mrs. Benedict's hospital chart and x-ray folder. "I'll be in the hospital," I said. "If you have any questions, just ask one of the nurses to page me."

He thanked me graciously and went to read her file. He spent much of Sunday afternoon in MICU, examining Mrs. Benedict and reviewing the hospital record, then talking Dr. McAllister, Mr. Benedict, and me. In essence he agreed with our evaluation and plans. As far as he was concerned, she had a confirmed case of Guillain-Barré syndrome.

The consultant recognized his main job was to reassure Mr. Benedict about our diagnosis and medical management. He was not hired to educate him (or us) about GBS. But the lawyer in Mr. Benedict wanted his money's worth, and when they met in mid-afternoon, he questioned his consultant like a star witness. I was present by invitation, though only as a spectator.

The meeting in conference room was very cordial, even if the discussion at times sounded like a legal deposition. Dr. DeJong, for his part, gave the information asked for.

Mr. B. "Of people who get this condition, how many die from it?"

Dr. D. "Overall mortality is about three percent. That's in our experience and in other large series as well."

Mr. B. "What do the patients die of?"

Dr. D. "Three things, mainly. Heart disease, for one. This is usually associated with autonomic dysfunction, such as arrhythmia. Another cause of death is pulmonary embolus, which is when a blood clot breaks off from the legs and travels to the lungs. The clot comes from lying in bed so long. To some extent this can be prevented by giving small doses of heparin. I should add that her doctors have given this treatment all along."

At the mention of "her doctors," Mr. Benedict gave a slow and approving nod.

Dr. D. "The third major cause of death in our patients is infection, such as pneumonia or septicemia. So far there seems to be no evidence for any of these problems in Mrs. Benedict."

Mr. B. "Is there any way to prevent the other two complications, the heart disease and infection?"

Dr. D. "Only by good care and catching the problems when they arise. One area of our research is the autonomic heart problem. So far, we haven't found a way to predict who will develop it or why. That's why it's so important to watch GBS patients closely, so you can treat the blood pressure crisis or arrhythmia as soon as they occur. Mrs. Benedict had one such crisis two days ago, and it looks like she came out of it okay."

Mr. D. "But you agree with the plasmapheresis therapy?"

Dr. D. "Oh, absolutely. Apart from time, it's the only effective treatment we can offer these patients."

Mr. B. "If this was your wife, would you do anything different? Anything at all?"

Dr. D. "Mr. Benedict, if this was my wife I would not change a thing. And if my wife happened to be in this hospital, with this condition, I would not transfer her to New York. I would leave her right where she is."

* * *

The first week in MICU, Naomi could only move her eyes, eyelids, and some facial muscles. She managed a weak smile but was unable to open her mouth wide or turn her head. Even so, Mr. Benedict decided the children should see their mother. His story about "infection" was wearing thin, and the kids, a six-year-old boy and ten-year-old girl, began to wonder out loud if Mommy was dead.

I was ambivalent about the kids seeing their mother paralyzed. They last saw her the morning of hospitalization. A visit when she was still paralyzed could help or hurt her situation, and I wasn't sure which. I suggested to Julian that he seek Naomi's opinion and he agreed. To his question, "Naomi, do you want the kids to come here?" she vigorously moved her eyes up and down: Yes!

Arrangements were made for the afternoon of March 14, her seventh day in MICU. The night before the visit, Julian tried to prepare the children, by explaining that Mommy was too weak to move and would not be able to talk, but that she loved them very much, and that she would come home faster if they let her know how much they loved and missed her.

About an hour before the scheduled visit, nurses tied Mrs. Benedict's hair back in a bun and attached a pretty red ribbon. They also applied a small amount of makeup to her lips and cheeks. With the head of her bed raised to 45 degrees, Naomi was sitting almost upright. Her head was buoyed by a pillow and turned to the left, so that she faced the side where her kids would stand. The tracheostomy tube and connecting hoses were covered discreetly with a bed sheet. By this date, the feeding tube had been removed from her nose, and instead placed through a small incision in her abdomen, leading directly to the stomach. From a distance, Mrs. Benedict looked almost normal, like someone sitting up in bed watching television.

Shortly after 4 p.m. Mr. Benedict and the kids arrived. Both children were smartly dressed in school clothes. By pre-arrangement, Julian took them straight to her room without any introductions to me or the staff. Worried about another autonomic surge, I discreetly stood in one corner of the room where she could not see me. The family entered and walked to her bedside.

"Hi, honey," said Julian. "I have Kevin and Cynthia with me."

Naomi managed a weak smile, an idiot-like grin the kids had never seen before. I saw it from across the room and shivered. Kevin and Cynthia just stood there, staring at their mother. For a few seconds—it seemed a lot longer—no one said anything. I wondered: Did we make a mistake, letting them see her like this?

"Hi, Mom," said Cynthia, a thin and pretty ten-year-old. I could tell she was destined to be a beauty like her mother. "Hurry up and get well, Mommy. We sure miss you. Daddy's taking good care of us."

"Mommy, this is for you," Kevin said, and he showed her an 8 x 11-inch picture he had drawn for the occasion. It displayed a red stick figure on a brown stick bed, above which were green block letters proclaiming GET WELL MOM SOON.

I sensed Mrs. Benedict wanted to smile and laugh and say what a wonderful picture it was, but all she could manage was the same feeble grin. Kevin didn't understand.

"Mommy, don't you like my picture? Mommy, why don't you hug me? I miss you Mommy!" He started to cry.

Cynthia nudged her brother and whispered sternly. "Kevin, Mommy can't hug you. She can't move right now."

The boy jumped away from Cynthia and tried to climb into his mother's bed. Julian pulled him back and he started to scream and cry louder. "MOMMY, MOMMY, MOMMY!"

Tears welled up in Naomi's eyes. I suddenly felt awful, and thought I might start crying also. What must she feel? How unfair! Why had we let them come in? I wanted to leave and let Julian handle this visit in his own way, but the cardiac monitor showed an accelerating heart rate. 110. 120. Then... 160.

Although we needed to treat her quickly, I spoke up without trying to sound alarmist. "Julian, I think we'll have to give her something. You better take them outside." He looked at me. and I pointed to the cardiac monitor.

"Let's go kids," he said, and ushered them out.

* * *

The next two weeks were dismal for the Benedicts. Lack of any clinical improvement was wearing Julian down. One telephone conversation after a plasmapheresis treatment on March 20:

"Hi Larry, any change?" (By then we were on a first name basis).

"Not yet, Julian. How are the kids?"

"Oh, they're fine. No permanent damage. They're just waiting for Mom to come home."

"I know. This is difficult for them. Well, tell them she will be home soon. And tell yourself that, too. It just takes time for the nerves to regenerate. If she remains stable, she should improve." Fortunately, there were no more autonomic crises, no more emotional upheavals. Just the paralysis. Day after day of paralysis.

Then a change. Twenty days and six plasmapheresis treatments after coming to the hospital, Mrs. Benedict began to move her *right index finger*. Regeneration!

"You're getting better," I told her. "You really are." We noted another big change: a broad, deep smile, far from the idiot grin displayed when her kids visited. I called Julian to relay the good news.

"How long will it take her to fully recover?" he asked.

"I don't know. Dr. McAllister says it could still take months, but at least nerve regeneration has started."

Without exercise, even the passive variety, paralyzed muscles develop disuse atrophy. Even after the nerve tissues regenerate, the muscles can remain severely weak. Since day one, we had provided range-of- motion exercises to Naomi's paralyzed limbs. Despite the exercises and tube feedings, there was some loss of muscle mass, and her weight was down twenty pounds at the end of three weeks. She needed more exercise.

From the Orthopedics Department, we arranged to borrow a mechanical exerciser, a machine that continually moves the leg or arm to help maintain muscle tone. The machine is used mainly to exercise limbs after orthopedic surgery, but we have also found it useful in some paralyzed patients.

Naomi had full sensation in her extremities, so we alerted her to possible pain. "This contraption will keep your muscles fit," I explained. "If it causes you any pain or discomfort, blink your eyes rapidly."

We secured her right leg to the exerciser. First the machine extended her leg. Then flexed it. Extended, flexed, extended, flexed. A full range of motion every twelve seconds. Fortunately, she felt no pain.

Naomi continued to improve, and by the end of March she could move her arms and head, but could not write or hold a glass. Also, her breathing muscles were still very weak. Normally, we can generate enough muscle strength to suck up a column of water to a height of about 100 centimeters (39 inches). People with respiratory failure from muscle weakness can suck up no than 20 centimeters (8 inches). The first time we tested her respiratory muscle strength, three days after the tracheostomy, Naomi managed only 10 centimeters of "sucking" pressure. Now it was up to 18 centimeters. Still low but increasing!

"You continue to improve," I said, "but we have to go a few more days before you can get off the machine. You'll make it. As soon as you do, we're going to throw a big party. If it's okay with you we'll keep it private. No one from the media will be invited." She smiled the equivalent of a hearty laugh.

We kept at it. Range-of-motion exercises. Tests of breathing strength.

Tube feedings. Constant monitoring. She had settled into MICU and seemed accepting of her new but very temporary home. The trauma of her kids' visit was ancient history.

To keep her mind occupied, Julian brought in cassette selections from Books on Tape, which she listened to through an ear plug. In two weeks, she went through Mark Twain's *Life On The Mississippi*, *The Cardinal of the Kremlin* by Tom Clancy, and *The Bonfire of the Vanities* by Tom Wolfe.

* * *

On April 12, her inspiratory force was 24 centimeters of water. We disconnected the ventilator and gave her supplemental oxygen through the tracheostomy tube. Now, for the first time in over a month, she was breathing entirely on her own. Since her inspiratory muscle strength was still suboptimal, I put her back on the ventilator after two hours.

"You did just great," I said, "but I don't want you to tire out. It's best if we do this a little bit each day. Tomorrow you'll go for four hours off the ventilator."

She moved her lips: "Where's my party?"

Naomi improved almost as rapidly as she had crashed. The next day, her inspiratory force was 30 centimeters. I took her off the ventilator with the understanding that she would be re-connected after four hours.

For three hours and forty-five minutes there was no sign of fatigue or respiratory distress. Encouraged, I told the nurses to leave her off the machine indefinitely, with the idea that she might go the whole night unassisted.

Fifteen minutes later Naomi asked to see me. She had recently regained some use of her writing hand and was now communicating with paper and pencil. She wrote BACK ON THE MACHINE?

"How do you feel?"

TIRED

I checked her respiratory rate, inspiratory force, cardiac rhythm, and blood pressure. They all pointed to one fact: physiologically, she didn't *need* the ventilator. Psychologically was another matter.

"Do you think you still need the breathing machine?" I asked.

YES

"Do you want to try and go without it a few more hours?"

NO

I have seen this response many times. Removing a patient from prolonged artificial ventilation often requires physiologic *and* psychologic adjustment. It makes sense. What has been critical life support is being discontinued; even though the patient no longer needs it, the "weaning" process takes time.

"OK," I said. "I think one more night. We'll put you back on the ventilator tonight. Tomorrow morning we'll disconnect it and let you go all day. If you do well during the day, you'll be able to go all night without it. I promise." She liked the plan.

On April 14, she went all day without needing or asking for the ventilator. And all night. On April 15, we had our party.

Follow-up

Naomi Benedict continued to recover muscle strength. She began swallowing food on April 18 and regained movement in her legs by April 21. On that date we removed her tracheostomy tube. On April 25, she was transferred out of intensive care to the hospital's rehabilitation unit.

As expected, she required extensive physical rehabilitation. On May 8, with the aid of a lightweight aluminum walker to keep balance, she took her first unassisted steps in two months. She went home from the hospital May 10.

Naomi continued muscle training exercises as an outpatient. Though progress was slow, she recovered completely. She started driving again in the middle of July and by September was back to a full schedule of meetings, parties, and charitable activities. She reported that Kevin and Cynthia were none the worse for her two-month absence and that life was back to normal.

The only scar from her ordeal is physical and small, where the tracheostomy tube entered her neck. She usually covers it with a high-collar blouse.

– END –

21. The Wild Man

Joe Cartney was one of our most difficult patients, and we almost lost him. He showed up in our emergency department—dumped there is more accurate—one cold Saturday morning. His brother or brother-in-law brought him in because Joe "was taken real sick all of a sudden." After imparting this message to one of the secretaries, Joe's relative sat him on a waiting room chair and went to "park the car." He did not return.

Left behind was a young man too sick to stay in any chair. He fell to the hard linoleum floor and proceeded to moan and wail. An ED nurse did a quick check of his vital signs, while asking lots of questions: "Who is this? Where'd he come from? What's his name?"

Only the hapless ED secretary had any information: "Mr. Joe Cartney... his brother or brother-in-law brought him in... said he's real sick, then left... said he'll be right back... didn't leave any phone number... didn't sign any forms."

As for the patient, all he could do was scream and flail his arms. Four of the staff lifted Mr. Cartney to a stretcher and brought him to the treatment area, then placed him in a bed. If he had a life-threatening condition, at least he was in the right place.

He could give no history worth a penny. He just moaned and screamed at the slightest provocation, calling for "Emma," presumably his wife or girlfriend, and various other people who he could not or would not identify. He knew his name but not the day, year, where he was, or how he got there. He could not answer any question coherently. He frequently resorted to profanity, like "you motherfucker." Joe Cartney was, in a word, delirious. Though acutely ill, he was simply unable to communicate his problem. The ED staff had no more history than a veterinarian presented with a sick dog found on the street. Methodically, the ED physician and nurse documented what they could.

Joe Cartney, Male, Age?
Vital signs. Blood pressure stable at 130/70; pulse irregular at 150 to 170 beats/minute (normal is less than 100/minute). Temperature 101 degrees.

Physical exam. Young male, medium build. Appears disheveled, unshaven, dirty. Skin moist and sweaty. No obvious signs of trauma or recent injury. Three tattoos noted: "Emma" over left arm, skull and cross bones over right arm, and "Born to die" over chest. Scars over abdomen, right thigh. ?knife wound. No neurologic defects, nothing to suggest he has suffered a stroke. Able to move all his extremities.

Cardiac rhythm. Irregular tachycardia. Appears supraventricular (not life-threatening)

Arterial blood gas test. Adequate oxygenation and ventilation (i.e., his lungs were working normally)

Other blood tests. Results pending, including "tox screen" (screen for toxins in his blood and urine, of drugs commonly used to overdose).

Chest x-ray. Neg. (Negative. No evidence for pneumonia).

For those first few minutes in the ED, Mr. Cartney didn't need cardio-pulmonary resuscitation or anything else heroic. He did need lots of attention, to keep him stable and in bed, to exchange his clothes for a hospital gown, and to find out what was ailing him. First guesses were acute alcoholic intoxication or withdrawal from alcohol, toxicity from illicit street drugs like PCP (phencyclidine, or "angel dust"), or some type of nervous system infection, either meningitis or brain abscess.

He did not carry the smell of alcohol. Nor did he appear yellow, bloated or wasted like an end-stage alcoholic. As for PCP, detection requires a urine measurement, ordered as part of the toxicity screen. In cases like this, until all the information is available, it is best to assume some type of drug overdose and manage accordingly. On that assumption, the ED physician placed a large, snake-like hollow tube through Mr. Cartney's nose and into his stomach. Through the tube she squirted some "activated charcoal," a highly absorbent black slurry that binds whatever pills or tablets it touches. After a few minutes the charcoal was sucked out of Mr. Cartney's stomach and with it, hopefully, any poisons he might have swallowed.

Of course, the ED team had no specific history for drug overdose, so other possible diagnoses were also considered. Like meningitis. Meningitis can be confirmed or excluded with a spinal tap and quick exam of spinal fluid under the microscope. But a spinal tap requires careful insertion of a thin needle in the patient's lower back, and Mr. Cartney could not stay still for that procedure. For the same reason a brain CT scan was not feasible, since it also requires a still patient.

And "still" he was not. Within twenty minutes of arrival he was referred to as the "wild man." To keep him in the bed, all four limbs were bound with leather restraints securely attached to the bed frame. Every minute or so he would try to sit up, pull against the restraints and bellow, "Get me out of here you motherfucker!" or some other profanity. Joe Cartney was a potential danger to himself, so he needed the restraints.

The ED's job is to treat emergencies and then triage, to make a proper disposition of the patient. This means treat and release, or treat and admit to the appropriate part of the hospital: intensive care, medical or surgical ward. Since the ED is on ground level, patients are either sent "upstairs" or discharged.

Acutely ill patients who pose a diagnostic dilemma, like Joe Cartney, may be kept in the ED for hours while tests are run and the problems sorted out. Does the patient need surgery? Admission to an intensive care unit? More tests in the ED? Joe Cartney was the epitome of diagnostic dilemma, but the ED staff did not wait for more tests. They sent him up to medical intensive care after only thirty minutes, probably a record for a patient not needing emergency surgery.

I was already in the ICU, making Saturday morning rounds, when the call came from the ED nurse. One of our ICU nurses answered the phone, took the message and hung up the receiver while announcing, "We have a wild one coming. A male."

"What's wrong with him?"

"They don't know. Possible overdose, possible meningitis. They just said he's wild and very sick."

Oh-oh.

* * *

Mr. Cartney arrived accompanied by two security officers, plus an ED nurse and physician. He was half sitting on the transport bed, bellowing and pulling on his restraints. A thick black tube stuck out of his nose, and I saw splotches of charcoal on his bed sheet and hospital gown.

The ED physician gave me a one-minute capsule history, finalizing her recitation with, "This guy's real sick, we don't know why, but he needs to be in MICU. Maybe an overdose, maybe meningitis, we don't know. There's nothing more we can do for him downstairs. He's all yours now."

We undid Mr. Cartney's restraints and transferred him to the ICU bed, then re-attached the leather straps. The ED and security folks promptly disappeared. As the MICU nurses went about their tasks, I moved to the head of the bed and looked at our new patient. He became eerily silent and stared back at me. He appeared to be in his late twenties. With eyes wide open, he did not seem to be in pain or even in any distress, which made me wonder, why all the wailing I heard about? The sweat on his brow, dilated pupils, and pulsating neck veins all gave the appearance of acute intoxication, but from what?

I tried a direct approach. "Mr. Cartney, what did you take?"

No answer.

"Did you take PCP?"

"Yes," he responded, slowly and in a low moan. His answer was not convincing, so I persisted.

"Did you take Alka Seltzer?"

"Yes."

"Did you take XYZ?"

"Yes."

We seldom ask yes or no questions, because you can't trust the answers, but this guy was not coherent and I thought it worth a try. Alas, he was not going to give any meaningful medical history.

Suddenly he grimaced and started yelling. "EMMMMA!"

"Mr. Cartney, who's Emma?" I asked.

He tried to sit up and only succeeded in pulling on his restraints. "Let me out of here!" he bellowed, then collapsed back to the bed.

His vital signs showed blood pressure 120/65, pulse irregular and ranging from 150 to 180 beats per minute, temperature 100.5. His electrocardiogram showed chaotic supraventricular rhythm, not immediately life threatening but definitely, severely, abnormal. Throughout all this activity we all wondered — what's wrong with him? What's the diagnosis here?

In another ten minutes we had more data. His tox screen was...negative. Neither the urine nor blood samples revealed any of several drugs commonly taken in overdose.

So PCP toxicity was, apparently, ruled out. Most of the other drugs tested for were analgesics, tranquilizers, sedatives and anti-epileptics. Obviously, not all drugs were tested for in the blood and urine screens, but we had to go with the information available. So to that point, we had no evidence for drug overdose.

Now we had to look for a treatable problem, like infection. As for his cardiac arrhythmia, it was clearly the result of some disorder and not the cause of his problems. His blood pressure was normal and he was not in shock. It was his fever and confusion that made meningitis and brain abscess a major concern.

Meningitis, infection of the membrane covering the brain and spinal cord, is a medical emergency. It can kill quickly, particularly when caused by some types of bacteria. Brain abscess is a pocket of pus inside the brain and also a very serious problem. Without surgical drainage of the pus, the patient will succumb.

Mr. Cartney was given a broad-spectrum antibiotic in the ED, in case he did have meningitis, but good practice mandated doing a spinal tap, so the spinal fluid can be cultured for any infecting organisms. There are too many different causes of meningitis to rely on empiric antibiotic therapy.

But we had the same problem as the ED staff. Mr. Cartney could not be safely positioned for us to place a needle in his spine. He was simply too combative. And his chaotic heart beat was a concern, even though he had a decent blood pressure. We were stumped. What to do?

More test results returned. His urine analysis was normal, no evidence for urine infection or diabetes. Kidney and liver function tests were normal except for a low serum potassium, a key electrolyte in the body's cells. Why a low potassium? Did he overdose on some diuretic medication that depletes the body of potassium?

And where was his family? Here was this fabulously ill guy, now in the hospital over ninety minutes, and no one around who knew anything about him. Where does he live? With whom? Who brought him in?

The information in the hospital's hastily-put-together chart was of no help. Phone number 999-999-9999. Social Security number 000-00-0000. Made me wonder, why not just "unknown" instead of nonsense numbers?

We called in a cardiology consultant, Dr. Sally Zingale. She was next door making rounds in the coronary care unit and came right over. Yes, she confirmed the heart rhythm was chaotic, a weird pattern of atrial tachycardia and atrial premature beats. And no, there was no specific treatment, at least not right then. She specifically did not recommend any anti-arrhythmic medication. "Find the underlying cause," she said. "I'll follow him along with you."

"Thanks," I replied, trying to sound sincere. In fact, I was frustrated. How are we going to figure this out?

* * *

So here was the situation. Mr. Cartney was sick, far sicker than any other patient I had that weekend, and we had no idea why, and no medical history. We suspected a drug overdose or nervous system infection. The tox screen was negative, and he was too combative to do a spinal tap. What next?

This dilemma was not handled in isolation. At any given moment I was consulting with two or three other physicians, including residents in training, plus the patient's ICU nurse and anyone else who would listen, so I had support. What I didn't have was a diagnosis.

Joyce Munson, one of the nurses, wondered: "Dr. Martin, what about rabies?"

"Rabies?"

"Yes, don't people with rabies act like this guy?"

"You mean wild and delusional?"

"Yes, just like our Mr. Cartney."

"Have you ever seen a case of rabies?" I asked.

"No, but I've seen it in the movies."

"Could be, Joyce, but I seriously doubt it," I said. "It would be the first case ever in this hospital, and it seems so improbable. From what I've read, rabies victims maintain muscle spasms constantly, especially the facial muscles. Mr. Cartney's grimacing comes and goes. He looks more like some type of drug toxicity. In any case, we've got to search for something treatable and rabies isn't treatable once a patient shows symptoms. But if we do the spinal tap, I'll save some fluid and check for the rabies virus, if nothing else turns up first."

"Okay. Just a thought," she replied.

Basically, I had two options. The first was to watch our patient in his current condition, see what happens over the next twenty-four hours, and wait for some more test results that were still pending — thyroid function, for example. Extremely over-active thyroid was a remote consideration. Another possibility was some drug toxin in his body that was being slowly excreted; if that was the cause, he might improve over time.

But what if the cause was a treatable infection, and we missed it? He could die for lack of the right antibiotics. So, the other option was to sedate and paralyze him with medication, then do the spinal tap and brain CT scan. This course of action would require connecting him to a breathing machine, since drug-induced paralysis stops all spontaneous breathing.

Death from meningitis, for want of a spinal tap and proper fluid cultures, seemed indefensible. With sedation we could control him, do the spinal tap, and maybe even figure out why his heart rhythm was so chaotic. On the other hand, intubation and artificial ventilation are not without hazard, and if there was a complication...

Jed Warner was with me, a top-flight senior medical resident. I respected his judgment.

"Jed, what do you think we should do?"

"Knock him out and ventilate him." Jed was a direct kind of guy.

"Just like that? But his breathing is okay. Don't you think that's a bit drastic? I mean, he's a little wild, but he doesn't require artificial ventilation for any of the usual reasons. His lungs are normal."

"I agree, Dr. Martin, but you're not going to get anything done with him. We can't do a spinal tap or CT scan. You can't even check a blood pressure measurement without full leather restraints."

"What if we have trouble intubating him? What if we paralyze him and the tube comes out of his throat? These things have happened. What if—"

"Obviously, anything can happen, Dr. Martin, but I don't know where we're going with this guy. He could improve, but he's got a low potassium, a chaotic rhythm, and he could also get worse. With either meningitis or some poison in his body, he could stop breathing on his own. Then where are we?"

Jed was right, of course. I just needed a little prodding to help make the decision. We therefore proceeded to paralyze and intubate Mr. Cartney. We asked the nurse to inject 2 mg of Versed (a sedating drug), followed by 2 mg of Pavulon (a paralyzing drug). All the while we monitored his heart rhythm. When Mr. Cartney was sufficiently relaxed, Jed proceeded with the intubation, which required placing a foot-long plastic tube into Mr. Cartney's trachea. Jed had experience with this procedure.

As Jed worked to insert the breathing tube, there was a sudden drop in Mr. Cartney's blood pressure. The reason was readily apparent from the cardiac monitor.

Another doctor in the room shouted, "He's in vee fib!"

I stared at the monitor in utter dismay. Ventricular fibrillation means the heart cannot pump out any blood. We had changed a chaotic *atrial* arrhythmia — one that provides a decent blood pressure—into a chaotic *ventricular* arrhythmia, called fibrillation. In ventricular fibrillation the heart's major pumping chambers, the ventricles, undulate like a bag of worms. In this state, they cannot pump out any blood. *None.* Uncorrected, ventricular fibrillation leads to brain death in about four minutes. It is one type of "cardiac arrest," a common cause of sudden death.

Already the nurses were setting up to defibrillate Mr. Cartney's heart.

I replied, trying to stay calm. "Is he being ventilated?"

"Yes, the tube's now in place," said my resident.

Only seconds had passed and I saw the paddles were in place, the defibrillator charged. "Stand back. Get ready."

Joyce pressed the buttons on the two defibrillator paddles straddling Mr. Cartney's chest. There was an audible "click" as 200 joules of energy surged through his heart. I remember thinking: *Damn. How did this happen? Are we going to lose him? Oh, damn. Damn, damn, damn. Please don't die.*

"I stared at the monitor. Okay, he's out of vee fib, back in a supraventricular rhythm. I see narrow complexes. Do we have a blood pressure?"

"One twenty by palpation," said one of the nurses.

"Start lidocaine. Let's give him a hundred milligrams."

Another minute passed. We all stared at the monitor.

"Jesus Christ! He's in vee fib again!"

"Shock him!"

"How much?"

"The full 350."

"Stand back."

He was defibrillated again, this time at the maximum energyl, 350 joules. Meanwhile, Jed continued to ventilate him with an AMBU bag. Mr. Cartney was too unstable to rely on a mechanical ventilator.

"Okay," I said, "he's back in some sort of regular rhythm. Please call cardiology again." A minute passed and Dr. Zingale entered the room. We handed her a bunch of long rhythm strips from the cardiac monitor. They documented the sequence of Mr. Cartney's alive-dead-alive-dead-alive cardiac rhythm.

"Vee fib," she said.

"I know, Sally. We shocked him out of it twice. I just gave him a bolus of lidocaine. Any other suggestions?"

"Do you have a blood gas and electrolytes?"

"They're cooking."

"Let's start him on a lidocaine drip at two milligrams a minute."

"Okay."

Arterial blood gas results returned and actually showed decent oxygen and carbon dioxide levels. And his potassium level was now normal, as he had received potassium replacement in the IV fluids.

Ventricular fibrillation did not return. We connected his endotracheal tube to the breathing machine. By now he was quiet, paralyzed from medication, and his heart was back to its previous chaotic, but at least life-sustaining, atrial arrhythmia.

We waited a half hour to make sure he remained stable, then did the spinal tap. The procedure went without a hitch. The fluid was clear. No sign of meningitis.

"Let's get him down for the CT scan," I said.

Four people wheeled Mr. Cartney and his machines to the CT scan in the basement. A half hour later we had the scan results. Normal. No brain abscess.

* * *

It was now two in the afternoon, some six hours after Mr. Cartney came to our ED. He was back in his room in the ICU and I had long since given up my afternoon plans out of the hospital. I sat staring at a mass of lab data and at his cardiac monitor. The answer was staring back at me, but I didn't see it. It was perhaps too obvious, I suppose, but there it was. Chaotic heart rhythm, delirious patient, low potassium level, no apparent infection. What did this man take that we had not measured or looked for? I worked with this substance all the time, yet inexplicably did not think of it until...

"Dr. Martin, his family's in the waiting room."

"What? Mr. Cartney's family?"

"Yes, they want to know if they can see him."

"See him? You bet. I'm going out to talk to them."

Dr. Warner and I went out to the waiting room. I was never more curious to meet a patient's family.

In the waiting room were two men and a woman. The men, like Mr. Cartney, appeared dirty and disheveled. They had grease in their hair, on their clothes. Perhaps, I thought, they just finished working in a gas station. And they smelled of cigarettes. But their appearance was not important. I needed *information.*

I introduced myself and Dr. Warner.

One of the men spoke. "This here is Joe's wife, Emma. How's he doing?"

The woman appeared to be about twenty-five. She wore no makeup and had that depression-era look: pallid face, faded dress, work style shoes. Reminded me of *The Grapes of Wrath.* She seemed both anxious and depressed at the same time. I felt sorry for the woman and not just because her husband was in a coma.

"He's in critical condition," I replied, "and we have no idea what's wrong with him. Who brought him in?"

"I did," replied the same man.

"Are you his brother? Why didn't you stay to give more information?"

"No. We're Emma's brothers," he said, and pointed to the other man, who didn't speak but gave a polite nod. "My name's Billy Echol. I brought him in. I was double parked, so I told the girl I got to go get Emma."

"Why didn't you return right away? We really have no idea what's happened to Mr. Cartney. Why didn't you at least call us?" I don't know why I gave this guy the third degree, but I was annoyed and couldn't help myself. My questioning didn't faze him.

"No phone, doc. And we had some car trouble. It's fixed now."

I was poised to ask numerous questions about Mr. Cartney. When did he get sick, what were his initial symptoms, is there any history of animal bites, any history of drug overdose, do they know if he took any pills, and so forth. I was expecting a difficult-to-get history with many blind alleys. But I was wrong. His brother-in-law headed me off.

"We found this in his room." He handed me a note, scribbled on the back on an envelope.

A note from Joe Cartney. *A suicide note!* In block letters, and crudely written, were the words:

EMMA. CANT GO ON ANYMOR.
BETTER WITH ME GON.
LOV, JOE

"Then he took something!" I was excited. We were getting close to an answer. "What did he take? Do you know what he took?"

Billy had that information also. He handed me a plastic pill bottle. "This here's Emma's asthma pills. It's empty. She says it was full yestiday."

I stared at the label. It was the missing piece of our puzzle.

> Emma Cartney.
> Theodur 300 mg, # 60
> Take 1 tablet twice a day with meals

Theodur. Brand name for *theophylline*. Of course! It all fit! Mr. Cartney overdosed on theophylline, a common asthma drug.

"Jed, let's get a stat theophylline level. Call the lab and tell them to please run it right away. After that, take Mrs. Cartney and her brothers in to see him. I'm going to call the kidney dialysis service."

I returned to the ICU and placed a call to Dr. Richard Malcolm, the physician on weekend call for the kidney dialysis. If Mr. Cartney took sixty tablets of Theodur, he may need hemoperfusion, a sophisticated technique that can wash out theophylline from the body. The process involves removing the patient's blood and passing it over a special column of charcoal that absorbs theophylline. The cleansed blood is then returned to the patient. Though highly effective, hemoperfusion is rarely performed. One reason is that it is only effective for some types of drugs, and the level has to be truly life threatening. Mr. Cartney's case checked both boxes.

When Mr. Cartney came under our care, theophylline was widely used to treat asthma. The Physician's Desk Reference of Prescription Drugs—the PDR—at the time listed over two dozen oral theophylline preparations, all for asthma and asthma-related conditions. In the twenty-first century theophylline is used much less frequently, and now outpatient asthma is mainly treated with inhalation drugs, which do not include theophylline.

For people who do take oral theophylline, mild toxicity is still fairly common. It happens to patients who take the drug as prescribed and, for one reason or another, build up a higher-than-expected level. In those situations, just stopping the drug is all the treatment needed.

Even patients who intentionally overdose with a theophylline preparation rarely need hemoperfusion. Usually the drug dissipates naturally in the body, and clinical improvement rapidly follows. But there is a limit to how much theophylline the body can tolerate. Mr. Cartney's case turned out to be the mother of all theophylline overdoses.

* * *

"I can't do hemoperfusion without a confirmed drug level," said Dr. Malcolm, now in the ICU and consulting on our patient.

"Richard, the theophylline level's being run now. This guy almost died twice on us already. The whole thing fits. Potassium goes down in theophylline overdoses. His cardiac disturbance is classic for theophylline toxicity. And his delirium fits the picture also."

"Why didn't you draw the level earlier?"

"We didn't think of it. It's not part of the routine tox screen, and we had absolutely no history. We're all smart in retrospect."

"When will it [the drug level] be back?" he asked. It was now 2:30.

"About three o'clock, the lab promised."

"Well, we're ready to go," Dr. Malcolm said. "My technician is warming up the equipment. If it is theophylline, how high do you think his level is? Do we know when he took the tablets?"

"No, his wife found him puking this morning. Her brother lives next door. He rushed him over here but gave absolutely no information. I guess no one did any looking around the house at first. Anyway, her brother just dropped him off in the ED and left. Then they found the note and the pill bottle. The way he's behaving, I'd say he swallowed the whole bottle around midnight. The pills were probably all dissolved into his blood by the time they pumped out his stomach this morning."

"So what do you think his level is?" Dr. Malcolm asked. The question was like, "So what do you think the final score will be?" I took up the challenge and called over to Jed, who was writing some chart notes.

"Hey, Jed, what do you think Mr. Cartney's theophylline level is?"

The therapeutic theophylline level — the amount in the blood that is supposed to help asthma patients when they take the pills as prescribed — is between 5 and 15 milligrams per liter, written 5-15 mg/L. Patients tend to get sick with nausea, diarrhea, or palpitations when the level exceeds 20. Above 30, the patient will likely be admitted to the hospital. Above 40, to the intensive care unit. Toxicology experts recommend hemoperfusion when the level exceeds 80. The highest level I had personally seen to this point was 84, and that patient had seizures.

"Oh," said Jed, "considering they've already pumped out his stomach, I'd say about sixty."

"Okay, let's write it down. Jed says sixty. I say eighty-five." I wrote both numbers on a piece of paper and put our initials by them. Then I said to Richard, "It's your turn."

"Oh, I don't know," he replied. "You see more theophylline toxicity than I do. We did hemoperfusion on a guy last year with a level of eighty-four [the same patient mentioned above]. He was pretty sick too, and he had seizures. I'll go way out and say ninety for this patient."

I wrote down Dr. Malcolm's guess next to the other two. Our range was 60-90. Whoever was closest, it was clear we all suspected a very high level.

But not high enough.

A few minutes later the ICU secretary called out, "Doctor Martin, the lab's on the phone."

I took the receiver. "Yes?"

The lab technician sounded excited, and asked if the patient was still alive.

"Going for hemoperfusion," I replied. "Are you sure about the level?"

Run twice, he said, and he was sure. I thanked him and hung up the phone.

"Welllll?" Dr. Malcolm asked, "the winner is...?"

I deadpanned the answer. "One hundred and sixty seven."

* * *

The hemoperfusion went smoothly, as Mr. Cartney's blood was routed from the large femoral vein in his thigh, through the machine where it bathed the charcoal column, which then absorbed the theophylline. The cleansed blood was then returned to his body through the same vein. Quite an elegant process, really. We removed Mr. Cartney's stomach tube as it was now superfluous.

After four hours of hemoperfusion his theophylline level went down to 88 mg/L. After eight hours it was 56. At that level his heart rhythm miraculously returned to normal. We stopped the sedative medication and he began to wake up.

Twenty-four hours later, his theophylline level was 21 and he was fully awake. We disconnected the ventilator and pulled out his endotracheal tube. He seemed all better.

And he proved to be a nice guy. No more wild gyrations. No more foul language. He seemed both pleasant and contrite.

"What happened?" I asked.

"I don't know."

"Did you want to kill yourself?"

"Not really. We jist had some problems. I'm sorry now. I ain't going to do it again."

"How many pills did you take?"

"I don't know. The whole bottle, I guess. They was Emma's pills."

"You know you almost died?"

"I'm glad I didn't."

"We have to ask a psychiatrist to see you."

"Okay. I understand."

Emma and two other family members came in next. Everyone was smiling, happy. And we—the professional staff—were all greatly relieved.

Mr. Cartney had no health insurance. The psychiatrist found him to be clinically depressed, mainly over poor finances, lack of a job, and related woes. The entire family was on food stamps. He recommended Mr. Cartney go to a county mental health facility. He did not believe Mr. Cartney was in danger of hurting himself again, at least not any time soon.

The next day, three days after his arrival, we discharged Mr. Cartney to the recommended facility. There he received some brief outpatient counseling, was judged to be no longer suicidal by the county's psychiatrist, and was sent home.

* * *

A week later I presented Mr. Cartney's case at a medical conference. Highlights:

- Most cases of theophylline toxicity are unintentional, usually because patients take, or are prescribed, more theophylline than their body can metabolize.
- The first case report of hemoperfusion for theophylline toxicity dates to 1978. The patient, a 50-year-old woman, was taking Theodur for asthma while in the hospital. She developed refractory seizures when her theophylline level went to 46 mg/L. After 4 hours of hemoperfusion, her theophylline level was down to 15.4 and her seizures gradually abated.

However, she died two weeks later, of pneumonia.

- The highest theophylline level in any of the articles I reviewed was 210 mg/L. That patient died.
- Theophylline toxicity is the most common poisoning for which charcoal hemoperfusion is performed.
- The majority of patients with a theophylline level greater than 120 mg/L developed seizures, and over 50% of them died. It is unusual that with so high a level (167 mg/L), Mr. Cartney never showed any seizure activity.

Follow-up

About three months later, while making rounds in MICU, I was paged to the phone by Jed, my resident.

"Guess what, Dr. Martin? Mr. Joe Cartney, remember him? He was in the ED last night."

"Of course I remember him. Not another overdose?" As soon as I asked, I realized this could not be, or I would have heard about it in the ICU.

"No. No. He had a mild respiratory infection and just came in to get some antibiotics. He's actually doing okay. No major problems. I found out from one of the ED residents. Just thought you'd like the follow-up."

"Thanks, Jed."

Well, I thought, not bad for a man who almost died. Twice.

– END –

22. 'Lou Gehrig' Strikes Again

I had long anticipated a distress call from someone in the Miraly family. When it comes I am at home, sleeping.

"Dr. Martin, Mt. Sinai Hospital calling."

"Yes?"

"I have a Mr. Ernest Miraly on the phone. He says he needs to speak with you. Can I put him through?"

"Yes, go ahead."

Mr. Miraly has a hoarse, quiet voice. Even face to face, during many sessions with the Miralys, I sometimes have difficulty understanding him unless I watched his lips move.

"Please speak up, Mr. Miraly. I can hardly hear you."

"Dr. Martin, my wife Angela, she's having trouble."

"What kind of trouble? What's happening?"

"With her breathing. I don't know what to do."

"Is she awake? Can she talk?"

"No. I just called 9-1-1."

"You called 9-1-1? How long ago?"

"Just before I called you. What should I do?"

He has already done it. The emergency medical squad will be at their house in a few minutes. And then what? Surely Mr. Miraly has understood my explanations, my recommendations, these past several weeks. I have done everything possible to warn him of this inevitable crisis, but he is not prepared for the sheer horror of watching his wife die.

"Mr. Miraly, please make sure the ambulance takes her to Mt. Sinai Hospital. I'll meet you in the emergency department." I know that EMS will get there before me.

"Okay, Dr. Martin. You'll call and tell them we're coming?"

"Yes."

"Will she go back into intensive care?"

"That's up to you. We'll see." Then, as an afterthought I add, "And it's up to her."

I place a call to the ED and speak with the doctor on duty, Roger Stanton. I explain the case, tell him what to expect, and ask that he hold off intubating her, if feasible, at least until I get there. Driving in I ruminate about Angela Miraly, and how she came to be my patient.

* * *

Only two months earlier Mrs. Miraly had developed her first symptoms, an unsteadiness of gait, a slight slurring of speech, some weakness in her arms. These symptoms grew worse to the point she could no longer drive. Her doctor sent her to one of our staff neurologists, Edgar Mason. Edgar determined the likely diagnosis and recommended she be admitted to the hospital.

Edgar had found telltale "fasciculations," fine, involuntary tremors of her arm and facial muscles. Progressive muscle weakness and these tremors suggest a specific, terrifying disease, amyotrophic lateral sclerosis. In ALS, there is atrophy and scarring of the spinal column nerves that control voluntary muscles. This nerve degeneration, of entirely unknown cause, can affect all the body's skeletal muscles, the muscles we can control at will. Involuntary muscles, such as found in the heart and other internal organs, are not affected by ALS.

Could she have something else? Muscle weakness by itself could reflect a dozen different diagnoses, from toxic drug ingestion to occult cancer to chronic fatigue syndrome. But she had no history of serious illness, no travel to dangerous places, no drug use of any kind except post-menopausal estrogen, no history of depression, no evidence for cancer. As noted in her chart by the admitting resident: "First Mt. Sinai Hospital admission for this 57-year-old white female, who was healthy and well one month prior to admission when she first noted weakness in her arms . . ."

Healthy and well. Always on the thin side, about 110 lbs. and 5'4" tall, a non-smoker, non-drinker, never before hospitalized except for childbirth. Mother of two grown children, grandmother of four, Mrs. Miraly was in her middle-age prime when ALS struck. Until weakness deprived her, she spent most of her free time with church work and other charitable activities. In all respects the Miralys were a pair of solid citizens to whom self-abuse was as alien as infidelity, a situation that made her disease seem so undeserved—compared, say, to cirrhosis in an alcoholic or emphysema in a smoker.

On the second hospital day Mrs. Miraly choked on part of her lunch which, because of weakened swallowing muscles and a depressed cough reflex, went into her lungs. Because of weakened diaphragms— the principal muscles of breathing—she quickly developed shortness of breath. That's when she came to intensive care.

On arrival to the ICU, about an hour after the aspiration episode, she was turning blue from lack of oxygen, so we intubated her trachea and connected the endotracheal tube to a mechanical ventilator. Then we sucked food out of her lungs and started antibiotics. It took us about three days before we could remove the tube and take her "off" the breathing machine.

By that time Dr. Mason had confirmed the diagnosis as "unequivocal ALS." He noted that her ALS was running a particularly progressive course, as opposed to a slower, more indolent course that afflicts some victims. He asked that I take over her care as principal physician since "her problems will no doubt be mainly respiratory." He would continue to "consult as necessary."

What about treatment? Anything new? I asked. No, he said, nothing. Nothing new, nothing old.

So I inherited Mrs. Miraly's case by virtue of the disease's effect on her breathing, which remained fragile. Pulmonary function tests two days after extubation showed very diminished lung capacity, a result of weakened respiratory muscles.

I also took on the task of explaining what euphemistically might be called "the situation." Doing so was not pleasant because ALS runs an inevitably downhill course. It is progressive, no one ever recovers, and most people die within three years of diagnosis. Some patients can live longer with machine support (for breathing) and continuous nursing care (for feeding, bathing, cleaning, and turning). It is a pure muscle-nerve disease, sparing all sensory and mental functions. Fortunately, ALS is not common; each year it is diagnosed in about one of every 100,000 people.

ALS is popularly known as Lou Gehrig's Disease because the great Yankee first baseman's affliction with the disease occurred at the height of his career, and was widely publicized. He developed ALS when only 35, at the start of the 1939 baseball season and his 17th year in the majors. At first, no one knew what was wrong. Despite increasing dis-coordination and difficulty ambulating, he suited up for the early games that season. But he could not hit or field the ball. Was the record-holding Gehrig (for hitting and consecutive games played) in a slump? Was he goofing off? What was going on? In May, he traveled to the Mayo Clinic, where the diagnosis was made. At Gehrig's request, his doctor wrote a note for public release, explaining the diagnosis of ALS and why Gehrig would not be returning to the baseball. He became an instant hero. The Yankees retired his uniform, number 4, and honored him at a special Yankee Stadium celebration in July. Gehrig died less than two years later, on June 2, 1941.

No progress in treating ALS had been made in the 50-plus years since Gehrig's demise. I had no good news for the Miralys.

I attempted to explain the diagnosis and its ramifications. I did so at her bedside because I wanted her to be involved as much as possible in decision making. Since she tended to turn her head to the left, a result of some neck muscle weakness, I stood on her left side, next to Mr. Miraly. He stroked her hair while I spoke. She looked gaunt, older than 57, her hair white and stringy, cheeks sunken in, eyes wide open. It was a look, I thought, of fear and apprehension. It would have been easy to forgo discussing her future—I sensed she would never ask questions on her own—but I felt compelled to raise the issue as soon as she could respond. Events that had precipitated her ICU transfer could happen again, at any time.

"ALS is a progressive condition, Mrs. Miraly. Dr. Mason tells me it has already progressed quite a bit since your first symptoms a month ago. There may come a time when you can't breathe at all, without the breathing tube and a machine."

"When will that be, doctor?" she asked, without showing any anxiety about the question.

"No, dear," Mr. Miraly chimed in, "that's not going to happen, is it doctor?"

What? He didn't want to hear this.

"Well, it very well could, Mr. Miraly. ALS is a progressive condition, and unfortunately we can expect her muscles will get weaker over time and—."

He shook his head as if, perhaps, I was lying, or talking about some other patient. He wanted me to shut up and, for the time being, I did.

A day later she was out of intensive care, on a regular medical ward. I talked with them further. By this time she was eating again, but only pureed foods since she couldn't handle solids well at all. Mr. Miraly was constantly at her bedside.

"We should talk about what can happen with this condition," I said. "There could come a time when you won't be able to eat on your own, or breathe without a machine. When that happens we can place a feeding tube in your stomach, and a breathing tube in your throat like was done a few days ago. We can do these things for you, but that's how you will live. I don't think Mr. Miraly can care for you then, and it will mean going to some sort of long-term facility, a skilled nursing home."

I tried my best to be direct and unequivocal, but also kind. I wanted to explain and make myself available for anything they wished to know. (Doctors can, with body language alone, make it clear they don't have time for questions. When that happens, patients usually don't ask any.) I sat down, looked in her eyes as I spoke, and made no sign of wanting to leave the room.

I brought up the subject of "advance directives," decisions about what to do when the end comes. Would she want to be kept alive on a breathing machine? Some ALS patients opt for this. It can even be done at home, but requires round-the-clock nursing care. Others have asked to be let alone, to die naturally, and this can be handled at home as well, for example through hospice care.

Some people, given the choice, opt for machine living over the alternative, which is early death. And in the culture of American medicine—an amalgam of technology and litigation, of ethics and economics, of philosophy and common sense—the individual doctor is obliged to ask the dying patient: "What do *you* want?"

Ethicists can argue that withholding and withdrawing life support are morally identical actions, but they are not the ones at the bedside pulling out tubes. Morality aside, it is certainly easier never to put the tube in than to have to pull it out. Don't put the breathing tube in and the patient dies a natural death caused by no human hand. Remove the tube and the patient dies because you pulled it out.

Of course, a terminally ill patient has the right to demand no life support, including stopping it once begun. She can even demand it up front, using an advance directive. The most common advance directive is the living will, a legal document wherein you state what is wanted should you end up in a 'terminal condition' or a 'permanently vegetative state'. The latter condition is rare, but "terminal condition" is not; it applies to a broad canvas of disease states. Like beauty, "terminal" is in the eye of the beholder, a semantic conundrum that is the principal flaw of any living will.

To my mind Mrs. Miraly was terminal because she had an incurable, progressively downhill disease; she would die of ALS much sooner than predicted from her normal life expectancy, without *or* with machines. With a ventilator and the enormous support it would mandate, she could live perhaps a few miserable years. Without a ventilator, perhaps a few months, or less. We were lucky to get her extubated and off the ventilator after she choked on her lunch. However, her degree of muscle weakness made it clear that the next episode of respiratory failure would commit her to the machine *until she finally died.*

All this I explained to the Miralys six-seven weeks before that late-night phone call, and told them about living wills, which they had never executed. Over ten days in the hospital I talked with them numerous times. I also met with their son and daughter, who came from out of town and stayed several days. Having families of their own, they had to return home, but by that time they, and their parents, had learned much about ALS and what to expect.

Son and daughter agreed that their mother probably wouldn't want to be kept alive on a machine, but that "it was up to her." Mrs. Miraly never made any declarative statement herself. Mr. Miraly, for his part, would only listen politely. He told me they would think about the issue. In truth, he and Mrs. Miraly simply didn't want to commit one way or the other. We arranged for a hospital bed at home, plus nursing care during the day and a special diet of pureed foods, and discharged her from the hospital.

So now I was going to see her again, in a do-or-die situation, in the Emergency Department.

* * *

I pull the car up to doctor's parking behind the ED and rush in. It is about 1:00 a.m. and the place is quiet, maybe four or five patients are being seen. I ask the triage nurse Rebecca where my patient is located.

"Room five. Dr. Stanton's in there now." I can see the waiting area where Mr. Miraly is sitting but he can't see me. I go straight to room five.

Mrs. Miraly is lying on a hospital stretcher, her head turned to the left. An ED nurse is taking her vital signs and Dr. Stanton is listening to her lungs. She is pale, gaunt, ashen, diaphoretic, with sunken cheeks and fast breathing: all the ways to describe a patient acutely and chronically ill, perhaps even dying. She is at least fifteen pounds lighter than when I last saw her.

I introduce myself to Dr. Stanton and we shake hands. We have seen each other in the hospital but not formally met. He is in his early thirties, and I recall that he only recently finished the training program in Emergency Medicine. This makes him an attending physician, and as responsible for his area, the ED, as I am for mine, the ICU.

"Larry, we've just started some IV fluids," he says. "We've sent a blood gas and she just had a chest x-ray. She's only been here a few minutes. I think she's going to need intubation. What's the situation? She's only fifty-seven?"

He means: She looks a lot older than fifty-seven, maybe seventy-seven. He is probably thinking what's also going through my head: Do we intubate this young/old patient with known ALS, connect her to a breathing machine, and send her to intensive care? Or do we not intubate, and send her to a regular medical ward where she will be made comfortable, but surely die soon? Had I not called ahead she would have already been intubated, no doubt, but he has held off waiting for me. He feels responsible for her care at the moment, and wants to get the issue resolved. He doesn't want her to die in his ED. Above all he wants to do the right thing.

ED doctors are as sensitive to end-of-life issues as any group around. They deal with them frequently, and often under difficult circumstances such as the one now presented by Mrs. Miraly. When patients look like they're about to die, the ED doctors *act*. They are trained to save lives, and sometimes decisions have to be made before the proper documents or knowledgeable relatives can be located. This is why, frequently, nursing home patients dying a natural death end up getting intubated, even if the patient is ninety years old and terminal with cancer.

The ED is a way station and patients stay there only briefly. Invariably the resuscitated terminal patient is sent to the ICU, where a different set of doctors has to sort everything out.

The ethical ideal of an 'autonomous patient' making cogent end-of-life decisions is rare. Most patients—most people before they are patients in any sense of the word—do not make end-of-life decisions, set up advance directives, or even discuss the issue with loved ones. Why should they? People have been dying for millennia without making 'end-of-life' decisions. Why all the emphasis now?

The answer is twofold. First, because American medicine has the machines and the staff to manage them. In the last several decades, in this country at least, an infrastructure has developed to keep dying people alive at all costs. Not just acutely ill patients who will eventually recover, but the terminally ill who will not recover, who will die without ever getting "off" the machines. Machines to breathe the patient, dialyze the blood when the kidneys fail, and feed the stomach, machines that can extend the dying process for a long, long time. And not just machines, of course, but people to service them *and* care for the patients—most of whom remain in the hospital or end up in a nursing home.

The second reason for the relatively recent emphasis on "end-of-life" decisions is because the alternative is poor utilization of medical resources. Since the infrastructure to keep dying patients alive is widely available, and mostly paid for by third parties, it often ends up being used when it should not be. "Should not be," of course, is a value judgment. Let's just say the machines are often used when neither the patient nor the family truly wants that level of care, and when the machines will not return the patient to any functional state.

Advance directives are supposed to help forestall inappropriate end-of-life care, but they are largely ineffective. Too few people execute them, and even then the wording is simply too general to be of much help. I can't recall a single instance where a living will was, by itself, sufficient to achieve any ethical decision. No matter what is written before hand, end-of life decisions always come down to a concurrent discussion with available family, the patient if he or she is able to participate, and the professional staff's outlook or prognosis. These decisions, once a patient is hospitalized, are complicated, often messy and fraught with anxiety. Contrary to what one might think, living wills do not make the doctor's task any easier.

* * *

"Yes, she's fifty-seven, Roger. And I honestly don't know the situation. I've talked to them frequently about this happening from ALS, told them what to expect, but they haven't made any decision yet."

"How are they leaning?" he asks. "Because I think we have to decide one way or the other, and soon."

"I know. Let me talk to Mr. Miraly again. I'll take responsibility for this."

"Okay, Larry. Let me know what you decide."

Roger leaves to see someone else in the ED, and I move to the bedside to examine Mrs. Miraly more closely. I listen to her heart and lungs, check her abdomen, review the chest x-ray. Everything points to pneumonia in one lung, presumably from aspiration; her muscles are too weak to allow her to cough and clear secretions, and these secretions have become infected. It is a common scenario.

Rebecca comes in with her blood gas results. They confirm respiratory failure (her CO_2 level is very high) and the need for intubation and a ventilator if she is to have any chance of survival.

I look at my patient and ask, "Mrs. Miraly, do you recognize me?" hoping for at least a head nod. She stares past me, unable even to make eye contact.

"Can you hear me?"

She does not respond. Covering her face is a loose fitting, lucent green oxygen mask. The mask hisses quietly. The only other sounds are her own breathing, and the beep-beep-beep of her oxygen monitor. Her cognition is gone and she can no longer participate in end-of-life decisions. I chance that, in the next few minutes at least, she will not completely stop breathing, and I go out to meet with Mr. Miraly. This time I would rather talk to him away from her bedside.

* * *

"Mr. Miraly, your wife is getting worse. She is dying," I tell him. "If we intubate her, put that tube in her throat like she had last month, she will end up on the breathing machine the rest of her life. You know we talked about this possibility. Did she make any decision about this? Did you two ever discuss it?"

There is no answer. His face is weary, eyes slightly bloodshot. He has a large bushy mustache and a full head of black hair, which make him look younger than his wife, even before she became ill. I have time to study his face since he only stares at me after my questions, as if I had another one to follow.

I don't. After perhaps half a minute he responds with a non sequitur in that low, almost inaudible voice. "She was a beautiful woman, Doctor Martin. A beautiful woman. You didn't know Angela. Where did this come from, this Lou Gehrig disease? What did she do wrong? She doesn't drink, she doesn't smoke. Why should she live connected to any machine? But how can I let her die like this?"

"It may be best to go this way, Mr. Miraly. Most patients with this disease die of pneumonia, and perhaps that is the best way. We can give her antibiotics and make her comfortable, and sedate her so she doesn't feel short of breath, so she won't feel any pain."

He shows me a picture taken ten years ago, of the two of them at a wedding. In the photo she is thin and pretty and they are both smiling, happy. The thought enters my head that I don't know these people at all, only her disease, and how it is destroying her body.

"Did you talk to your children about this, I mean about making this type of decision?"

"They don't know she's here now. I don't want to call them now. It's two in the morning." He has not answered my question, so I guess the answer is no.

"Mr. Miraly, should we make her DNR [do not resuscitate], and just treat her with antibiotics and no intubation? Is that what she would want us to do? Or does she want to live on the breathing machine?"

"I don't know. What do you think we should do?"

"Mr. Miraly, we've talked about this before. It's not my decision. I think you have to understand the options. She'll die if we don't put the tube in, but if we do and she recovers from this pneumonia, she will remain on the breathing machine. Then she'll be bedridden, but alert. We'll have to do a tracheostomy to put the breathing tube in her neck, and place a feeding tube into her stomach. She'll need a nursing home. And she'll die eventually, with all these tubes. You need to realize this is how it will be. Is this what she would have wanted? You said she didn't want to live like that?"

"I don't know," he mumbles.

"Did you talk about it with her, at all?"

"No, I don't think so."

I remain silent. After another long pause he says, "Doctor, these last few weeks have not been good to her. I don't have my Angela anymore. Do whatever you think is best."

I suddenly appreciate he is no longer involved, and I am getting nowhere. Somewhat surprisingly, he has not asked to see her in the treatment room. He knows she is yet alive, and I assume he is fearful of what he'll see; he can no longer deal with what has happened to them. For different reasons, patient *and* husband are each incapable of making end-of-life decisions. If words alone are important, I can obtain any answer I wish to hear. By posing questions a certain way I can get him to mouth words, but they will be without conviction. Realistically, there is no reason to continue this dialog. I am at the point where IT IS UP TO ME. Let her die of natural causes, humanely, or subject her to machines, tubes, life support for as long as her body can hold out.

"Then I'll decide, is that what you want Mr. Miraly? Do you want for me to decide?"

"Yes, you decide, doctor. Do what's best, doctor, please."

The waiting room is virtually empty, and we are sitting side by side on a long row of hard plastic seats. I need a witness and call Rebecca over; for the moment she is not busy. Apart from registering Mrs. Miraly upon arrival, Rebecca does not know her problem in any detail; a different ED nurse is providing care as I speak with Mr. Miraly. Rebecca sits down on another seat directly opposite us. She is young, in her late twenties. She has worked as triage nurse in the ED for about a year. I don't know if she has ever been involved in end-of-life discussions—I doubt it, at least while a triage nurse—but she is a professional and I just need someone to listen in. I briefly explain Mrs. Miraly's condition, and our conversation, then resume my questioning.

"Mr. Miraly, I want this nurse to hear you, because this is very important. You understand your wife is dying of a terminal condition?"

He looks at me and nods yes.

"She has never stated her wishes, of what to do when the end comes, is that right?"

He looks at Rebecca, then me, and again nods yes.

"Because she has a terminal condition, if I think it's best to just keep her comfortable, and not to place her on life support machines, not to put a tube into her throat, then you go along with that, Mr. Miraly?"

He forsakes the nod and says, "Yes, if that's for the best."

So it's okay, then, Mr. Miraly, *not* to put Mrs. Miraly on life support machines? Not to intubate her throat and connect her to a ventilator?"

"Yes, if that's what's best for her." Did he emphasize the "if"? I seek to clarify further.

"You understand that we'll keep her comfortable, make sure she doesn't suffer, and that she'll still be cared for in the hospital until the very end?"

"Yes, if that's what you think is best," he whispers. There is no emphasis on "if," no emphasis on "best," no emphasis on anything. He is staring at her photo, and is no longer looking at me or the nurse. I ask Rebecca if she heard everything, and if she has any questions for me or Mr. Miraly. This is not a deposition, only a conversation that I want witnessed. Rebecca affirms she heard him clearly and that she has no questions. I thank her and she returns to the triage desk.

The ED is quiet. In the distance I hear an ambulance siren, and closer in the muffled voice of the hospital operator paging a physician. I am thankful we are alone; no one is nearby, no one is observing us. I grab his free hand and hold it tight with both my hands. His hand is limp. His head is bowed and he is crying. I feel as though I could cry, too, but hold it back.

I envision us as posing in some modern tableau—two vulnerable people, patient's husband and doctor, one crying and one trying not to. If the scene was painted, perhaps by a modern-day Norman Rockwell, it could be titled "Decision Time in the Emergency Ward." We sit still for a full minute. No more words pass between us. His mind has retreated to some happier time long past. I am not so lucky. My mind is rooted in the present, the god-awful decision-time present. I search for precedents and realize there are none, at least none just like this. The disease may have an inevitable natural course, but every case is different, with singular nuances of family, doctor, hospital, and location in space and time. I think to myself: *We are all unique upon the earth; disease does not change this.*

I let go of his hand. He remains silent. I get up and walk toward Mrs. Miraly's room. On the way I glance back at Mr. Miraly. He is not watching me, only staring at his wife's picture.

My patient remains obtunded, her breathing fast and labored. At the moment, no one else is in the room. Fluid is dripping into her veins. I glance at the vital sign sheet. Her blood pressure and heart rate are holding up. I call Roger and Rebecca into the room, and go over my conversation with Mr. Miraly, and how he has agreed to do whatever I think is right for his wife. I explain how difficult this has been for both of us, and what my decision is. They nod approval.

And then I intubate her.

Comment

One might wish for a sophisticated medical or ethical explanation for the decision made that night, but there is none. It was simply a decision made in the heat of the moment. The same patient, in a different setting, or with a different physician, or accompanied by all her family and not just her husband, might well have come to a different result. At *that* moment in time, in *that* situation, intubation just seemed the right thing to do. Mrs. Miraly lasted another week on the ventilator, without any resolution of her pneumonia. Before she succumbed to her illness, the family made her "Do Not Resuscitate," so that when the time came we did not attempt CPR.

– END –

23. "Shock Him!"

John Capowski, 51, came to the hospital for an altogether different problem than what brought me to his bedside. He showed up in our emergency room weak and lethargic, with a three day history of nausea, vomiting and diarrhea. He came because he couldn't keep anything down, and also because it was the middle of the night and Mrs. Capowski was afraid. She insisted he see a doctor and drove him to our ER. They arrived about 1 a.m.

The previous day he had missed work, calling in sick to the car plant where he worked as assembly line foreman; the line makes engine blocks for several car models. His job was not difficult, he liked the work and was seldom absent. A second day absent, though, and he would have seen a company doctor, if for no other reason than a return-to-work note. He rarely saw his own physician, certainly not for anything routine. And he wouldn't think of calling his doctor at midnight, so the ER was a convenient choice.

To the ER physician on duty Mr. Capowski did not seem acutely ill. Vital signs were normal, although his blood pressure was slightly on the low side. But vital signs like blood pressure and heart rate are not the whole picture. Despite his size, a muscular 5'11", 210 lbs., he appeared wan and listless, sick enough to warrant further investigation. Vomiting and diarrhea can deplete the body of electrolytes and the only way to know for sure is to measure the blood levels. And who would want to tell Mrs. Capowski to take him home? She hovered over him with an air of insistence: 'do something'.

Sure enough, Mr. Capowski had a low blood sodium and potassium, meaning he had lost a significant amount of electrolytes. He needed hospitalization, a recommendation as much to his chagrin as to his wife's relief. Other tests in the ER, including chest x-ray and EKG, were normal, so he was admitted with the diagnosis "Probable viral syndrome, dehydration, hyponatremia [low sodium], hypokalemia [low potassium]." The plan on admission was "fluid replacement and monitoring of electrolytes." The ER doctor started an intravenous solution of sodium and potassium and sent him to the ward.

Mr. Capowski reached Tower 9 about 5 a.m. Four hours in the ER is not a particularly long delay, especially since treatment was started there. By the time of transfer he was feeling much better. The night shift nurse on Tower 9 noted he was "stable . . . not short of breath" and "has no complaints."

From then until 8 a.m. things went well. Mr. Capowski slept a little, made one call to the nurse for an extra pillow, and otherwise created no stir. Shortly after 8 a.m., he got up to go to the bathroom and halfway there slumped to the floor. A nurse in the hallway, Nancy Whitehead, heard a crashing sound— probably the IV pole hitting the floor along with the patient—and went in to check. She found Mr. Capowski on the floor, unresponsive, face down. She tried to arouse him. Nothing. She instinctively felt for his carotid pulse. Nothing.

One second he was standing, breathing, living. A few seconds later, no heartbeat, no respirations, a lifeless hunk on the floor.

* * *

People die suddenly and non-traumatically all the time, several hundred thousand a year in this country alone. It usually comes from cardiac arrest; the heart suddenly stops beating, followed immediately by cessation of breathing. Sometimes a rescue squad arrives in time to revive the victim, but far more often there is nothing to revive when help does come; the heart is irreversibly gone and Mr. Jones or Ms. Smith is "dead on arrival" to the closest hospital. Sudden death from cardiac arrest happens to people at work, on the golf course, in airplanes, at shopping centers, at home. It can happen while exercising, sitting or sleeping. Usually the victims are older and have some history of heart disease, but many are younger (less than 50) and have no known heart problem.

Basic Cardiopulmonary Resuscitation (CPR) has been a staple of Red Cross teaching for decades. It is taught in schools, churches, office buildings, basically any place people will gather for a two hour session. The lessons are simple. Come upon a victim? Establish unresponsiveness by shaking him or her. Without this crucial first step, you may give CPR to someone merely napping. Unresponsive? Immediately call 911 or tell someone to do so. If another person is with you, also have that person get an AED (Automatic External Defibrillator) if one is in the area.

Check for breathing and pulse. If not certain, provide 30 compressions over the lower breast plate (sternum) with the heels of your hands. Then give two mouth-to-mouth breaths, followed by 30 more pumps. Repeat the sequence (two breaths, 30 pumps) until there is a pulse and breathing, or you become exhausted, or help arrives.

There are some dramatic saves with basic CPR but the technique is, by itself, not sufficient for the true cardiac arrest victim. Chest pumping and mouth breathing provide a fraction of normal heart and lung function, and can only be sustained for minutes. So CPR's main value is in buying time until people can come with advanced life support equipment. But if the rescue squad doesn't arrive quickly the situation is hopeless. Or worse. The heart rhythm may return too late, leaving the victim alive but severely brain damaged, a human vegetable relegated to institutional care. It happens.

No doubt in some cases the heart may be ready to quit, and a resuscitation attempt is futile. The organ may be so diseased that any measure is bound to fail. But for most sudden death victims there is probably much life left in the ticker *if only it could be re-started before the brain is damaged.*

A dead car battery means a dead car, but if the battery only needs to be jump-started the car might be able to go another 100,000 miles. Without energizing the battery no amount of gas or engine repair will give life to the car. Of course, car batteries can be dead a long time before coming to life again; in cardiac arrest the victim has, on the outside, only 4-5 minutes. After that, brain damage from lack of oxygen is irreversible (with rare exceptions, such as after near-drowning in cold water).

There is another difference between the heart in cardiac arrest and a dead car battery. To understand what happens in most sudden death cases, accept the fact that the heart doesn't just shut down; it begins to violently *wiggle* for a few minutes, *then* shuts down. Only during those precious few minutes *before* total standstill does the victim have a chance.

The heart is an amazing bundle of muscle and nerve fibers. These fibers, distributed in discrete bundles throughout the organ, have automaticity, which means they fire off automatically until the end of life. You can't move an arm unless your brain sends a signal to the arm nerves to move the arm muscles, but your heart muscle will contract whether you think about it or not. Nerves bundles in the heart are not controlled by the brain.

Each firing of the cardiac nerves causes one contraction or heartbeat, and with it the heart muscle pumps blood out the aorta, to the rest of the body. The adult human heart beats about 70-80 times a minute for the life of its owner; this comes to 37-42 million heart beats a year, or *billions* of beats over the average life span.

Most cases of cardiac arrest occur because the heart's nervous system suddenly runs amok. The cardiac rhythm changes from regular to a *chaotic, purposeless wiggling* called *ventricular fibrillation*. In anyone not ready to die, not expected to die, ventricular fibrillation is the most feared diagnosis imaginable. From the onset of VF, the victim becomes instantly unconscious; in only a few minutes the heart in VF will stop all activity and be forever motionless. A totally motionless heart is called asystole, literally absence of systole or contraction of the heart. The fibrillating heart can be resuscitated; the heart that fibrillates and then goes into asystole is beyond hope (with rare exception).

The chaotic nerve firing of ventricular fibrillation emanates from the ventricles, the large pumping chambers of the heart. VF is not to be confused with the relatively benign rhythm *atrial* fibrillation, a common malady in older people. In AF the smaller chambers (atria) fibrillate but the ventricles beat normally. People can live for years with AF; no one can live more than a few minutes with VF.

The heart's visual appearance in ventricular fibrillation has been likened to a bag of worms. In VF every heart muscle fiber beats to its own rhythm without regard to the one adjacent; there is no coordination, no synergy, no *pumping action*. As a result, no blood leaves the heart during ventricular fibrillation and there is no pulse. Sudden death is not always from VF but VF always means sudden death) unless it is quickly reversed.

Why does a heart suddenly go into VF? Heart attack is probably the most common reason: a sudden lack of blood supply to a critical part of the heart tissue. People who die of "heart attack" usually have VF first, then die.

But lack of blood supply can also manifest as a non-fatal *arrhythmia* or abnormal beating of the heart. Not surprisingly, many cardiac arrest victims have a history of arrhythmia in the preceding months or years. Fortunately the converse is not true; most cardiac arrhythmias, which are exceedingly common, do not presage VF.

Here's what a heart with normal cardiac rhythm sounds like; each thump represents one heart beat.

**thump--------thump--------thump--------thump--------thump--------
thump--------thump--------thump**

A too-fast heart beat is called tachycardia. It can be regular or irregular. Here's the sound of a regular tachycardia.

**thump-thump-thump-thump-thump-thump-thump-thump-thump-
thump-thump-thump-thump**

Here's a tachycardia where every third beat is abnormal, called trigeminy.

**thump-thump-THUMP-thump-thump-THUMP-thump-thump-
THUMP-thump-thump-THUMP-thump-thump-THUMP**

And a tachycardia where the abnormal heart beats are different from each other *and* occur at irregular intervals:

**thump-thump-THUMP-thump-THUMP----thump-thump-thump---
thump-*THUMP*---THUMP-thump-thump-thump-THUMP**

There are many variations in tachycardia and its opposite, bradycardia, or slow heartbeat. However, as long as there is a "thump," some blood will be pushed out of the ventricles to the rest of the body. Treatment of arrhythmias depends on the nature of the thumps—diagnosed by the EKG and physical exam—and how the patient feels. Treatment is usually required if the patient experiences discomfort ("palpitations") or the abnormal "thumps" pump too little blood to the body. In any case, doctors have one basic rule: treat the patient, not just the arrhythmia. Sometimes cardiac arrhythmias are best left alone.

VF is never best left alone, unless death is expected. There is no "thump" in the VF heart, no pulse, because the heart wiggles without purpose. If reversal doesn't come within minutes the patient always dies.

The only way to recognize VF is with an EKG machine or other type of cardiac rhythm monitor. These machines, which connect to the patient via wires, sense the heart's electrical activity and provide a continuous tracing of the cardiac rhythm. Given such a device, diagnosis of VF is not usually difficult. In fact the biggest obstacle to recognition is probably artifact, from electrical noise. This noise can be generated by the environment or by wires improperly attached to the patient. It can sometimes look like VF. When the victim is without pulse or respirations, the rescuer focuses on checking for VF and making sure the wires are properly attached.

Figure 1 shows a normal heart rhythm taken from an EKG tracing; each narrow, symmetrical spike or deflection is preceded and followed by shorter, rounded deflections; taken together, the three deflections represent the electrical activity of *one* normal heart beat (one "thump"). The distance between the tall spikes in this tracing indicates a heart rate of about 70 beats/minute. The closer the spikes are to each other the faster the heart beat. Note in this tracing how every heart beat looks the same.

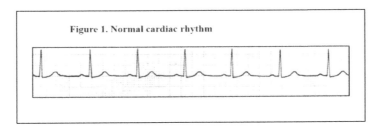

Figure 1. Normal cardiac rhythm

The cardiac rhythms shown in Figures 2-5 are all abnormal. Each rhythm represents one of the following diagnoses (not in order):

- regular tachycardia
- asystole
- rhythm where every second beat is abnormal (bigeminy)
- ventricular fibrillation (Mr. Capowski's rhythm).

Which is which? Try to answer before proceeding (answers at end).

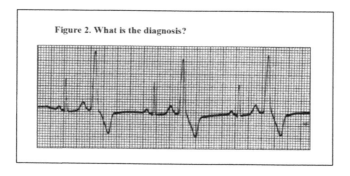

Figure 2. What is the diagnosis?

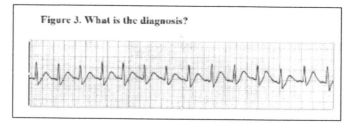

Figure 3. What is the diagnosis?

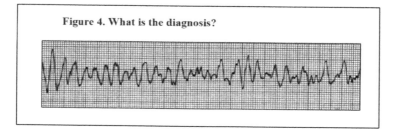

Figure 4. What is the diagnosis?

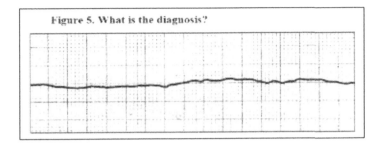

Figure 5. What is the diagnosis?

The only therapy for VF is *defibrillation*, literally a jolt of direct current electricity delivered through the chest. This jolt doesn't actually re-start the heart like a car battery; instead it stuns the heart momentarily, stops the VF, and allows the heart's normal nerve firing to resume. Defibrillation requires a machine, called a defibrillator, that can be attached to the victim via wires to deliver the shock. But where do you find a defibrillator outside the hospital?

The answer is: lots of places. Defibrillators for public use are AEDs, or automatic external defibrillators. In the several decades since Mr. Capowski was cared for in our hospital, there has been a sea-change in public awareness of CPR, and in placement of AEDs in millions of public locations: schools, airports, shopping centers, sports arenas, office buildings—generally, wherever people congregate. AED-training is also now incorporated into basic CPR courses, but even without training they are easy to use.

There are several Youtube videos on use of AED. Below are links to two videos, with a screen shot from each. As the second Youtube video emphasizes with a bar graph, speed of defibrillation is critical.

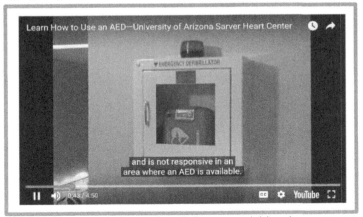

https://heart.arizona.edu/heart-health/learn-cpr/video-how-use-aed

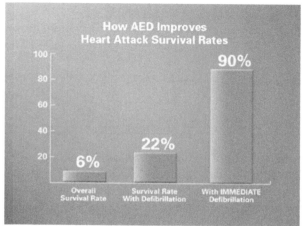

https://www.youtube.com/watch?v=xfvu5FCQs6o

AEDs are now so automatic that people without special training can use them (see pictures below).

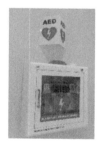

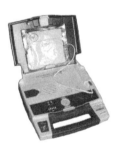

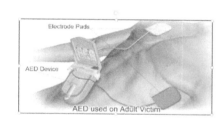

AED in Wall   AED unit   AED paddle placement

Step 1: Access the AED. Step 2. Open it. Step 3. Press a button to activate it. Step 4. Follow the voice prompts. Many lives have been saved with AEDs. Without defibrillation, most cardiac arrest victims have little chance of survival. With AED's, many can be saved.

* * *

Nancy ran into the hallway and yelled: "Call a chest team!" Chest team is our code for cardiac arrest. Different hospitals use different codes, such as "Dr. Heart!" and "Code Blue!"

The ward secretary punched a special 3-digit number into her phone and the hospital operator instantly answered, "Where?"

"Tower nine."

Elapsed time since Mr. Capowski's fall: 30 seconds. Nancy grabbed the red crash cart standing in the hallway as the loudspeaker boomed:

"CHEST TEAM TOWER NINE. CHEST TEAM TOWER NINE. CHEST TEAM TOWER NINE. CHEST TEAM TOWER NINE."

I heard it. Everyone did, because chest team is broadcast hospital-wide as a signal for specific people to come, wherever they are: the anesthesiologist to intubate the patient, the senior medical resident to help manage the arrest, the respiratory therapist to set up the ventilator, and all doctors in the immediate vicinity. This time I am in the vicinity, three rooms away seeing another patient. I go into the hallway and immediately see all the tumult.

As I enter Mr. Capowski's room there are already two nurses and two medical residents, initiating resuscitation maneuvers. Mr. Capowski has been turned over and is now supine on the hard linoleum floor. Elapsed time from fall: 45 seconds. Nancy is pumping on Mr. Capowski's chest, while one of the residents is pushing air into his mouth and nose with a bag-mask-valve contraption called an AMBU bag. These devices are safer and more effective than mouth to mouth breathing, and so are universally used by professional rescuers. Another nurse is hooking up monitor leads from the defibrillator, which now sits on the floor next to the victim. The other resident is feeling for a pulse.

"What happened?" I ask. A dumb question, as everyone is in the midst of resuscitation. The man arrested. That's what happened.

"I just came on," says Nancy, while pumping. "This is Mr. Capowski. He was admitted a few hours ago with dehydration. I was told he was stable. He just collapsed."

"Do we have any history?"

The night intern who admitted him to the ward is apparently not here. Probably signed off and taking a shower. Another resident, who entered right after me, begins reading through the medical chart out loud. "He came in just this morning. Let's see, no history of heart disease. Taking no heart or other meds. In fact, pretty much no medical history. He works in a factory. Smokes a pack a day, for 30 years. Drinks alcohol socially. His sodium's low, 129, K [potassium] is only 3.3. They gave him some K in the ER. His EKG was read as unremarkable in the emergency room."

"Let me see it." His EKG is in the chart and it looks normal. I begin to grasp the picture. Mr. Capowski wasn't expected to die. This is not terminal cancer or end-stage heart disease.

"He's in vee fib!" yells the nurse who attached the chest leads. She instinctively reaches for the defibrillator paddles to apply to his chest.

Time from fall: one minute 40 seconds. We are on a roll. Most in-hospital chest teams take at least a couple of minutes for someone to bring the defibrillator to the bedside *and* attach the leads *and* read the monitor rhythm. Time is life and, so far, this is good time.

Meanwhile, Nancy is still pumping and the resident is still AMBU bagging. More people enter the room—too many, in fact. "Chest team" always brings in too many people. Better too many than too few, but sometimes crowding is a problem. Everyone who enters has a question or a suggestion of some sort: Where's the oxygen? Does he have an IV? How long's he been down?

Nancy, sensing impending chaos, quickly turns her head to me and without hesitation intones, "Dr. Martin, you're in charge."

Me in charge? I just walked in, and for a minute have sort of just stood by while others do the work. Why am I in charge? Of course, resuscitation by a bunch of people requires someone be in charge; otherwise conflicting orders tend to be yelled by many lieutenants. And, someone has to be ready to make perhaps the most important decision of all: when to stop.

The person trained in Advanced Cardiac Life Support is usually in charge. So-called ACLS incorporates defibrillation and use of cardiac medications. Trained, of course, means simply having taken the American Heart Association's two-day ACLS course and knowing what to do. Any of the medical residents could be in charge, since I am no more knowledgeable in ACLS than they are, but to quibble at this point is self-defeating. Nancy is going by the book and wants to establish a leader, and I understand. My thoughts on this matter take about three seconds.

I notice the paddles are now applied to his chest. We do not use an AED, where in essence the machine assumes the bystander knows little to nothing about resuscitation, and so makes all the decisions. Hospitals use a defibrillator that requires making decisions, giving orders.

"Okay, give him 200 joules," I say. Joules are the energy units for electric countershock. In ventricular fibrillation (VF) we start with 200 joules, and if that doesn't work go to 300 joules and if that doesn't work, 360 joules.

"Stand back! Hands off!" yells the nurse holding the paddles.

Rescuers have to keep hands off the patient and all equipment touching the patient, or they can be shocked by the defibrillator energy. So CPR always stops when the shock is delivered—at that moment there is no pumping on the chest, no bagging. Hands touch the shocking paddles only: one held against the upper right chest beneath the clavicle and the other pressed under the left nipple, over the heart. Buttons on both paddle handles are pressed simultaneously and the jolt of electricity is delivered to and through the victim's heart.

The buttons are pressed, the jolt delivered. Zap! Mr. Capowski's body jerks. All eyes turn to the defibrillator monitor. Nothing seems to have changed. The monitor shows he's still in VF. Time elapsed: two minutes 20 seconds.

The anesthesiologist walks in, along with the respiratory therapist. There are now a dozen or so people in the room. Only five or six are needed, tops; the anesthesiologist is one of them. Observing that the shock has done nothing, she asks if we want her to intubate the patient. Placing an endotracheal tube in his throat would certainly allow for better ventilation and oxygenation than using a face mask.

Intubate now or shock again? The decision is easy. There is a universal algorithm for treating VF, taught as part of ACLS. The thinking about VF goes like this. Only electrical defibrillation will correct the problem; nothing else seems to work. Two hundred joules frequently does the job, but sometimes only a higher dose will work when the lower dose fails. Also, repeat shocks seem to work better even when the dose is kept the same. Any delay in providing shocks can be fatal. Therefore, don't waste time trying to intubate. Even in the best of hands it could take a minute. Just give the initial shocks. *First thing to do is give three successive shocks: 200-300-360 joules.* Do this before any drugs are given, before an attempt at intubation, even before placing an intravenous line.

"No, he needs another shock," I respond. "Go to 300 joules." The defibrillator knob is turned a notch to 300.

"Everyone off." The paddles are applied against his chest.

Zap! His body jerks again.

"Let's check the rhythm." Still VF. Three minutes 10 seconds have elapsed. Nancy bends down to resume chest pumping but I tell her to hold off.

"Give him 360." This is the maximum. If he doesn't respond, then we'll resume CPR, go to intubation, IV epinephrine and another shock at 360. Then more epinephrine and another 360. On and on. The longer he goes without responding the less likely he'll recover.

Zap!

One-two-three seconds. The VF rhythm disappears and we have . . . a flat line! Asystole! But before I can yell for something else to try the flat line is interrupted by regular blips.

"We have a rhythm!"

Again, all eyes are on the monitor. In the space of ten seconds the chaotic wiggling of VF has changed to asystole and then to a regular heartbeat. Not a normal rhythm to be sure, but one that *gives a pulse*. We can feel it in his groin. He is still unconscious, but he has a pulse and a blood pressure. Now I let the anesthesiologist to intubate him.

* * *

An hour later he is in the intensive care unit, under my care. And he is waking up! Mrs. Capowski is at his bedside. She had been called by a nurse during the resuscitation, told her husband had "suddenly collapsed" and "the doctors are working on him."

We have much work to do on our new patient but she needs to be with him, now. Who knows what the next 24 hours will bring? His heart could stop again and he could die next time. We are all a bit uneasy. I have asked a cardiologist to see him right away, and help us determine where to go next; I assume he will need cardiac catheterization as soon as possible. Considering he was unconscious for less than four minutes, and his heart was manually compressed during some of that period, Mr. Capowski has an excellent chance of being mentally fine.

I am smug, for this was truly a miraculous save. A combination of luck and nursing skill. In fact, it is one of the very few times I have been witness to a successful in-hospital cardiac arrest outside the intensive care unit or emergency department. In-hospital resuscitation is usually dismal for several reasons. First, people who develop VF on a hospital ward are typically elderly and/or debilitated and/or with a terminal disease.

Successful chest teams in the setting of advanced disease are rarely happy events, even when the patient survives. Hospitals routinely resuscitate chronically ill, debilitated patients but save very few; most die later, during the same hospital stay. Survivors who leave the hospital are usually relegated to long-term nursing home care, often connected to a breathing machine.

Another reason for dismal outcome has to do with patient location. In the ICU patients are monitored continuously whereas on the regular medical ward, only every few hours. Thus, a patient can go into cardiac arrest *without anyone aware*. It is not at all unusual for a nurse or orderly to come upon a patient pulseless and cold.

A third reason is response time. Even when the arrest is promptly identified it may take several minutes to get the crash cart and attach the defibrillator wires. In non-patient care areas, such as the waiting rooms, parking garage, hospital lobby—all places patients have arrested—resuscitation can take much longer. AEDs are often placed in these remote areas, to be used by anyone.

Mr. Capowski's luck was in falling where he did and someone hearing him fall, immediately, someone who was trained in what to do and able to do it without hesitation. The chest team worked like it's supposed to.

* * *

In the ICU, Mr. Capowski's post-arrest EKG showed evidence for a myocardial infarction, a heart attack, no doubt sustained while walking to the bathroom. Most likely his smoking and the low electrolytes, plus some type of underlying heart disease, all contributed to VF. Because of VF he did require emergency cardiac catheterization, carried out the same afternoon. The cardiologist found a critical narrowing in one coronary artery, and they were able to open it up with balloon angioplasty. During the procedure he received intravenous lidocaine to prevent recurrence of VF. Also, a heart surgeon was available in case angioplasty failed and coronary bypass became necessary. Fortunately, it didn't.

Mr. Capowski left the hospital just four days later, on his own feet. By then at least six different doctors and nurses had regaled him about the event, including me. I emphasized prevention. "You know your heart stopped, it could happen again, you really have to quit smoking."

Other hospital personnel commented in awe, hinting at his miraculous recovery. "Do you remember anything that happened? Did you feel anything?" And others were simply clinical and direct. "Your heart stopped due to a coronary blockage; the artery is open now but you must stay on this [heart drug] indefinitely. We'll see you in the office in three weeks."

Bestselling books have been written about near death happenings, the experience often framed in religious and mystical overtones. But to Mr. Capowski, he might as well have been merely sleeping. He remembers nothing from the time he got out of bed on Tower Nine until he woke up in the ICU. He is not particularly religious, and shrugs off all the attention with a "that's-my-fifteen-minutes-of-fame" kind of attitude. He had glimpse of neither heaven nor hell, and admitted to no "experience." As for any lasting effects, Mrs. Capowski swears her husband has the same low key, taciturn personality he had before hospital admission.

Was Mr. Capowski resuscitated from death or near death? During resuscitation was he sleeping or unconscious or dead? Questions like these can make you glassy-eyed with metaphysical thoughts. From a pure physiology perspective, all that happened is his heart stopped pumping. During this period his brain had sufficient oxygen, due to basic CPR, so that he suffered no loss of cerebral function.

The day of discharge I went in to say goodbye. By then, "your heart stopped" was almost a cliché, and I didn't bring it up. It was clearly on his mind, though. Not because he planned to write a book but because, I suspect, he was plotting out his post-hospital life style.

"Doc, my heart really stopped that day?"

"Yes, it did."

"I'll be damned. I feel great now."

– END –

Answers to cardiac rhythm questions

Figure 2. bigeminy

Figure 3. regular tachycardia

Figure 4. ventricular fibrillation

Figure 5. asystole

Glossary

AED – automatic external defibrillator.

AIDS - acquired immunodeficiency syndrome; in AIDS, the body's infection-fighting immune system is severely depressed and altered. AIDS is caused by the human immunodeficiency virus (HIV).

angiogram - a test whereby dye is injected into a blood vessel to outline the vessel and any abnormality within it. See pulmonary angiogram.

apnea - absence of breathing; an apneic episode or spell is a short interval of not breathing.

arterial - pertaining to the arteries, e.g., arterial blood.

arterial blood gas - refers to the pressure of oxygen and/or carbon dioxide in arterial blood; abbreviated ABG. An "ABG" test routinely measures pressures of both gases, along with the level of blood acidity.

arterial line - a thin tube inserted into a patient's artery, usually the radial artery, for purposes of monitoring blood pressure or drawing frequent arterial blood gases. This technique is only used in intensive care units or in the operating room.

artery - blood vessel that carries oxygen-rich blood from the heart to the body's organs and tissues.

artificial ventilation - method of supplementing or taking over a patient's breathing with a machine (ventilator). The patient is connected to the ventilator via an endotracheal tube inserted through the mouth or nose.

artificial ventilator - see ventilator.

autoimmune diseases - a large and heterogeneous group of diseases characterized by altered immunity; usually, antibodies form in the blood directed against some part of healthy tissue.

bigeminy - cardiac rhythm where every second heartbeat is abnormal.

biopsy - removal of a piece of tissue from some part of the body for diagnosis.

blood gases - general term for carbon dioxide and oxygen in the blood; see arterial blood gas.

bronchitis - inflammation or infection of the airways (bronchi).

bronchodilator - a drug that relaxes airway smooth muscle and helps open up narrowed airways; useful in treating asthma.

bronchoscope - thin, flexible tube used to perform bronchoscopy; useful to diagnose many pulmonary conditions.

bronchoscopy - procedure whereby a thin, flexible tube (the bronchoscope) is inserted, via the mouth or nose, into the lungs; used to visualize the airways and diagnose many lung diseases. A biopsy can be done through the bronchoscope.

capillary - the smallest blood vessel. Capillaries go to all organs to bring vital oxygen and take up carbon dioxide; in the lungs the process is reversed: fresh oxygen is taken up and carbon dioxide excreted.

carbon dioxide - colorless, odorless gas, a byproduct of normal metabolism; abbreviated CO_2. Carbon dioxide is excreted by the lungs through the natural process of ventilation.

catheter - a thin, plastic tube that can be inserted into part of the body, such as a blood vessel or the bladder.

catheterization - general term for inserting a tube into a blood vessel. In cardiac catheterization a thin tube (catheter) is inserted through a vein or artery and into the chambers of the heart.

CO_2 - chemical symbol for carbon dioxide, a product of metabolism that is largely excreted by the lungs during breathing

coronary - pertaining to blood vessels that serve the heart muscle; so-called because the coronary vessels encircle the heart like a corona.

coronary care unit - area of hospital for patients with acute heart disease, including suspected or diagnosed heart attack.

CPR - Cardiopulmonary resuscitation, the series of steps done to revive a person who has stopped breathing and/or whose heart has stopped beating

CT scan - Computerized tomography scan (also sometimes called CAT scan for computerized axial tomography); a sophisticated x-ray technique which can "slice" any section of the body to reveal details of anatomy not seen with conventional x-rays.

coumadin - a medication that makes the blood less likely to clot; used to treat many medical conditions, including pulmonary embolism; can only be taken by mouth.

defibrillator - machine that can provide an electrical shock to the heart in order to convert the cardiac rhythm to normal.

dialysis - process of cleansing the blood of toxins; in *hemo*dialysis, used to treat kidney failure, blood is removed through a vein, passed through a special filter that removes the toxins, then returned to the patient.

diuretic - a drug that promotes urine flow; a diuretic can be taken by mouth as a pill or administered by the intravenous route.

DNR - Do Not Resuscitate, often written as an order in the chart of patients who are terminally ill.

dopamine - an intravenous drug used to raise a patient's low blood pressure. See pressors.

dyspnea - shortness of breath.

ED – emergency department; this area of the hospital is also often called the ER or emergency room, but it is seldom is just one room.

emboli, embolism - when a blood clot moves from one part of the body to another; in pulmonary embolism, the clot moves from some region of the body to the lungs.

emphysema - a chronic pulmonary disease, usually due to smoking, that leads to shortness of breath and blockage of airflow.

encephalitis - inflammation of the brain; see encephalopathy.

encephalopathy - a general term for confusion due to global brain disease. There are many possible causes including inflammation (encephalitis) and lack of oxygen.

endoscopy - general term for insertion of a flexible, diagnostic tube (endoscope) into a hollow organ; gastrointestinal endoscopy involves inserting an endoscope into the stomach or intestines.

endotracheal tube - a hollow plastic tube, approximately a foot long and a centimeter in diameter, inserted through the mouth or nose and into the trachea. It is used to facilitate artificial ventilation.

ER – see ED.

esophagus - hollow tube that connects the mouth with the stomach.

exsanguinate - to bleed out, hemorrhage.

gastroenterology - specialty of medicine involved with diagnosing and treating gastrointestinal (stomach and intestinal) disorders; a specialist in this field is a gastroenterologist.

hematocrit - percentage of blood volume comprised of red blood cells (oxygen-carrying cells); normal range for hematocrit is 38-45 percent in women, 42-50 percent in men.

hemodialysis - see dialysis.

hemoptysis - coughing up blood.

heparin - a medication that makes the blood less likely to clot; used to treat many medical conditions, including pulmonary embolism; is given intravenously or subcutaneously.

HIV - human immunodeficiency virus, the virus responsible for causing AIDS.

housestaff - the interns and residents in a teaching hospital; also spelled house staff.

hyperthyroid - elevated level of thyroid hormone, the hormone that regulates metabolism.

hyperventilation - over-ventilation or over-breathing. Hyperventilation is accompanied by a reduced carbon dioxide level in the blood.

hypothyroid - low level of thyroid hormone.

hypoventilation - under-ventilation or under-breathing. Hypoventilation is always accompanied by an elevated carbon dioxide level in the blood.

hypoxemia - low oxygen level in the blood. Hypoxemia can manifest as either a low oxygen pressure (PO_2) or a low oxygen saturation; see PO_2.

immunosuppressed - when the body's immune system for fighting infection is suppressed or altered; this is the principal problem in AIDS patients. Immunosuppression is also found in many other situations, e.g., during treatment with cancer drugs.

insulin - a hormone made by the pancreas, necessary to allow glucose to enter the cells; a lack of insulin leads to diabetes.

insult - in medical terminology, refers to damage or injury to a part of the body, e.g., an insult to the liver.

intern – a physician in the first year of training after graduation from medical school; see also "resident."

intravenous - route for medication or fluids given directly into a vein.

intubation - the placement of an endotracheal tube into the patient's airway, usually for purposes of providing artificial ventilation; see artificial ventilation.

meningitis - inflammation of the meninges, the thin membrane that covers the brain and spinal cord.

MICU - medical intensive care unit; area of the hospital for acutely ill patients, excluding those with surgical problems or primary cardiac disease.

Munchausen - name given to a patient who fakes illness in order to gain medical attention or admission to the hospital; after Baron von Munchausen, an eighteenth-century teller of tall tales.

mycoplasma - a bacteria-like organism that can cause pneumonia.

O_2 - chemical symbol for oxygen, vital for life. We bring in oxygen through breathing.

opportunistic infection - an infection by an uncommon organism (may be a bacteria, virus, or fungus), one that takes advantage of a patient's suppressed or altered immunity (hence opportunistic), such as is found in AIDS patients.

overdose - general term for taking an excess of medication; an overdose can be intentional (e.g., suicidal), or accidental (e.g., swallowing too many pills for headache relief).

oxygen - essential element of life; a colorless, odorless gas that comprises 21 percent of earth's atmosphere. Abbreviated O_2.

Pickwickian syndrome - term used to characterize a patient who is obese, falls asleep easily during the day, and has an elevated level of blood carbon dioxide.

plasmapheresis - technique of separating out certain proteins from the plasma. Plasmapheresis is used to treat Guillain-Barré syndrome and other illnesses.

pneumonia - infection of the lung tissues; can arise from many different types of micro-organisms, e.g., bacteria and viruses.

PO_2 - Partial pressure of oxygen (O_2) in the blood. Any value for PO_2 above 60 is usually considered a safe level; lower than 60 indicates hypoxemia and potential danger for the patient.

pressors - intravenous drugs used to support or raise a low blood pressure. One commonly used pressor is dopamine.

psychosis - severe mental disturbance characterized by personality disintegration or some loss of contact with reality; schizophrenia is one form of psychosis.

pulmonary - referring to the lungs.

pulmonary angiogram - dye is injected into the main pulmonary through a catheter, to outline the arteries within the lungs; this test is occasionally used to help diagnose pulmonary emboli.

pulmonary embolism - see emboli.

resident - refers to doctor in training, after internship.

respiration - general term for the process of bringing in oxygen from the atmosphere to the blood and excreting carbon dioxide from the blood to the atmosphere. Respiration is made possible by the process of breathing.

respirator - see ventilator.

respiratory failure - condition where the lungs have failed in their primary function of bringing adequate oxygen to the blood and of excreting carbon dioxide; in respiratory failure, the level of blood oxygen is either reduced or the level of carbon dioxide is increased, or both.

scan - a general term for a variety of tests that "scan" or survey a part of the body, usually done in the radiology department. A lung scan is done to look for pulmonary emboli.

sepsis - infection involving the blood stream.

subcutaneous - under the skin; a subcutaneous injection is one given just under the skin, into the subcutaneous tissue.

surgical intensive care unit - area of hospital for patients who need intensive care after an operation (e.g., after heart surgery), or patients who have suffered major trauma (e.g., gunshot wound). (Compare with MICU, coronary care unit.)

tachycardia - fast heart rate, usually over 100 beats per minute.

TB - see tuberculosis.

teratogenic - able to cause birth defects.

trachea - medical name for "windpipe," the airway that connects the back of the throat to the lungs. The trachea is the largest airway and divides into two bronchi.

tracheostomy - a surgical procedure that places a hole in the trachea, through which is inserted a short (usually plastic) tube. Tracheostomy is almost always done on patients who need long-term artificial ventilation.

trigeminy - cardiac rhythm where every third heartbeat is abnormal.

tuberculosis - disease caused by a bacteria called *mycobacteria tuberculosis*; abbreviated TB. TB usually involves the lungs but may also appear in any part of the body.

vasoconstrictor - any substance that constricts or narrows blood vessels.

vein - blood vessel that carries venous blood from the tissues back to the heart; venous blood is low in oxygen. See arterial.

venous - pertaining to the veins, e.g., venous blood.

ventilation - a general term for the physiologic process of delivering fresh air to the lungs for gas exchange. The term is sometimes used interchangeably with respiration.

ventilator - a machine capable of taking over a patient's breathing, also called a respirator. See artificial ventilation.

ventricular fibrillation - abnormal heart rhythm where the heart's ventricles "fibrillates" and so cannot pump blood out to the body; left uncorrected, it is always fatal.

Also by Lawrence Martin, M.D.

Consenting Adults Only

A novel of medicine, mayhem and a vicious love triangle in modern-day Las Vegas

The novel's protagonist is Las Vegas Emergency Medicine physician Dr. Joshua Luvkin, a nice, upstanding guy from the Midwest – with a few problems.

- He falls in love with nurse Barbara Wilson, which leads to his breaking up with girlfriend Dr. Judy Berkowitz, also an emergency medicine physician. Barbara moves in. Judy shows up. What ensues is remindful of *Fatal Attraction*.
- He meets Jack Strawn, an obese guy who enters quickie weight reduction contests, aka The Biggest Loser, but via a bathroom break and not from dieting. This somehow leads to Dr. Luvkin's investment in a Las Vegas cable porn show…and more publicity than he ever wanted.
- He is sued for malpractice, as if he didn't have enough trouble already. Will he settle? Go to trial?

Consenting Adults Only brings together Dr. Martin's experience in medicine and medico-legal issues to portray a young physician besieged by unpredictable people and unintended consequences.

Available in print and as ebook on Amazon.com

From a 5-star Amazon review:
"I loved the book! It's got everything…doctors, lawyers, crooks, malpractice, stalking, Las Vegas…and a surprise ending I'm not going to spoil. If you read it on a plane, you're going to have your neighbors reading over your shoulder. Get ready for that."

The Wall: Chronicle of a Scuba Trial

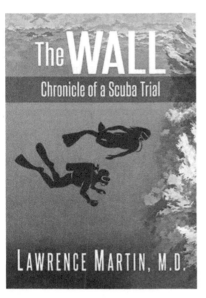

A young woman is lost on a scuba dive in Grand Cayman. Did she suffer nitrogen narcosis? Or did she commit suicide? Experts argue both scenarios in a civil trial that takes place 14 months later. Her parents are the plaintiffs. The defendants are a large corporation and its dive master on that fateful day. There are several experts called to testify, including the author. The two lawyers object to each other's arguments, cite precedent, drill their experts. Yet one thing is missing: her body. It will never be recovered. The Wall is fiction but it reads like a real case. Put yourself in the jury box, listen to the experts and lawyers battle it out, then make your decision along with the jury. How will you decide? For the plaintiffs or the defense?

Available as ebook on Amazon.com

From a 5-star Amazon review:
"**Great Reading.** An entertaining account of a trial following the tragic death of a young woman diving in the Cayman Islands. The author intertwines scuba, medical and legal issues deftly. He obviously knows them all well. He presents plaintiff and defense arguments skillfully and leaves you wondering until the very last sentence. I won't spoil the surprise but I love the unusual way the author ends the book.